MW01120608

Trans and Sexuality

Grounded in cutting-edge qualitative research, *Trans and Sexuality* explores the sexuality of people who do not identify with the gender that they were assigned at birth. Arguing that whilst splitting members of the trans community into distinct groups might seem like a reasonable theoretical procedure, the pervasive assumption that group membership impacts on the sexuality of trans people has unduly biased opinions in this highly contested, yet dramatically under-researched, area. Moreover, whilst existing literature has taken a purely positivistic standpoint, or relies on methodology that could be seen as exploitative towards trans people, Richards is careful to place the real-life experiences of trans research participants at the heart of the work.

Showing that sexuality extends beyond the bedroom, this forward-thinking book touches on topics such as identity, sexuality, and the intersections between the two. Richards takes a cross-disciplinary approach and considers the sexuality of trans people within the contexts of psychiatric and psychological settings, including Gender Identity Clinics, as well as in the broader contexts of cultural and community settings. The implications of the research at hand are also explored with respect to counselling psychology and existentialist philosophy.

Trans and Sexuality will appeal to academics, researchers, and postgraduate students in the fields of gender and sexuality, counselling, sociology, psychotherapy, psychology and psychiatry. It will be of particular interest to those seeking an in-depth and up-to-date overview of ethics and methodologies with people from marginalised sexualities and genders.

Dr. Christina Richards BSc (Hons), MSc, DCPsych, CPsychol, MBACP (Accred.), AFBPsS is an HCPC Registered Doctor of Counselling Psychology, Chair Elect of the Division of Counselling Psychology, and an Associate Fellow of the British Psychological Society (BPS). She is also an accredited psychotherapist with the British Association for Counselling and Psychotherapy (BACP). She represents the East Midlands to NHS England's Clinical Reference Group (CRG) on Gender Identity Services, and is one of the few psychologists recognised by HM Courts and Tribunals Service as a Specialist in the field of Gender Dysphoria, thus allowing her to prepare medical reports for the Gender Recognition Panel.

She is a Senior Specialist Psychology Associate at the Nottinghamshire Healthcare NHS Trust Gender Clinic and a Clinical Research Fellow at West London Mental Health NHS Trust (Charing Cross) Gender Clinic. She works in this capacity as an individual and group psychotherapist and psychologist conducting psychotherapy, assessment, and follow-up clinics as part of a multidisciplinary team, as well as conducting research, supervision, and service improvement plans. She lectures and publishes on trans, sexualities, and critical mental health – both within academia and to third-sector and statutory bodies; and is a co-founder of BiUK and co-author of the Bisexuality Report.

She is the Editor of the journal of the British Psychological Society's Division of Counselling Psychology: *Counselling Psychology Review*. Her own publications consist of various papers, reports, and book chapters and she is the co-author of the *BPS Guidelines and Literature Review for Counselling Sexual and Gender Minority Clients*; first author of a clinical guidebook on sexuality and gender published by Sage – Richards, C., & Barker, M. (2013). *Sexuality and gender for mental health professionals: A practical guide*. London: Sage; first editor of the *Palgrave Handbook of the psychology of sexuality and gender*; and is the first editor of a multidisciplinary book about people who identify outside of the gender binary of male or female – Richards, C., Bouman, W. P., & Barker, M. J. (2017). *Genderqueer and non-binary genders*. Basingstoke: Palgrave-Macmillan. She is also sole editor of Richards, C. (2017) *A view from the other side: Therapists' art and their internal worlds*. Monmouth: PCCS Books.

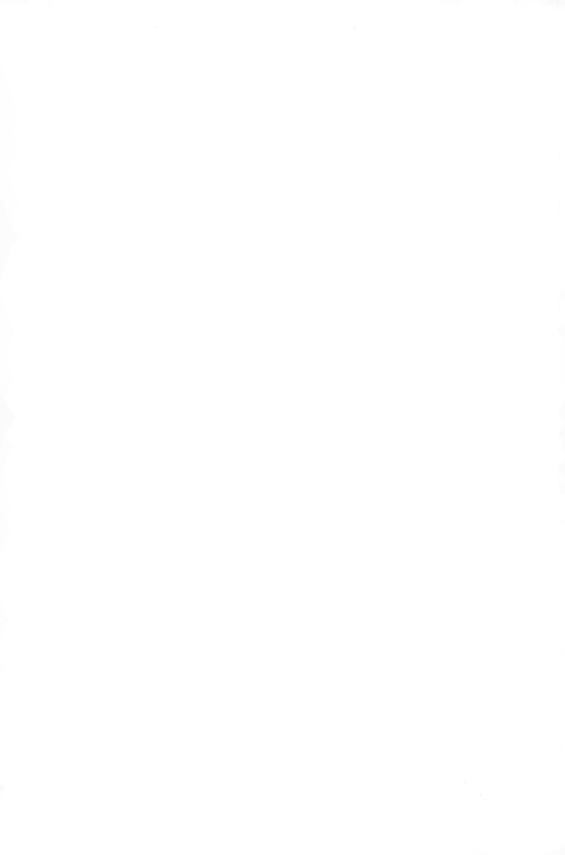

Explorations in Mental Health

For a full list of titles in this series, please visit www.routledge.com

Trans and Sexuality

An Existentially-Informed Enquiry with
Implications for Counselling Psychology

Dr. Christina Richards

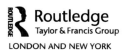
Routledge
Taylor & Francis Group
LONDON AND NEW YORK

First published 2018
by Routledge
2 Park Square, Milton Park, Abingdon, Oxon OX14 4RN

and by Routledge
711 Third Avenue, New York, NY 10017

Routledge is an imprint of the Taylor & Francis Group, an informa business

British Library Cataloguing-in-Publication Data
A catalogue record for this book is available from the British Library

Library of Congress Cataloging-in-Publication Data
A catalog record for this book has been requested

ISBN: 978-1-138-90356-2 (hbk)
ISBN: 978-1-315-69682-9 (ebk)

Typeset in Bembo
by Apex CoVantage, LLC

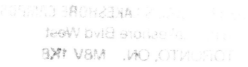

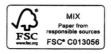
MIX
Paper from
responsible sources
FSC   FSC® C013056
www.fsc.org

Printed and bound in Great Britain by
TJ International Ltd, Padstow, Cornwall

When I think about how trans people are represented in terms of our sexuality we are very, very dehumanised.

(Mr Fox – a Participant)

This does represent . . . a confusion. But not a confusion for what I feel like and what how I see myself, but external society's assumptions about me, can just be too, too heavy sometimes and it's just . . . yeah psychologically it can be very demanding. That's it.

(Cee Cee – a Participant)

Contents

Acknowledgements

First, I would like to thank the participants for their invaluable contributions to this research. You have made me think, a lot, and have made me a more accomplished clinician and researcher for it. I would like to thank my doctoral supervisor Dr Peter Martin for his indefatigable advice, guidance, and support throughout the latter part of the doctoral thesis upon which this monograph is based – you are a model of kind, penetrating intelligence. I would also like to thank my examiners Professors Martin Milton and Simon DuPlock for an enjoyable and rigorous viva voce, and for their excellent suggestions for this monograph. All mistakes and omissions are naturally my own.

I would like to thank the Hans W Cohn scholarship for their financial support – too often necessary work is stymied by a lack of resources and so funds such as you provide make all the difference. I would especially like to thank: Phil for everything as ever – this is done because of you; Dr Meg-John Barker for their extraordinary support throughout the whole process; and Dr Penny Lenihan for support, advice, and not least for showing me how to actually be a counselling psychologist at the coalface of NHS practice. I would also like to thank Dr Rob Clucas for being a bloody nice chap; Dr Stuart Lorimer and Dr Leighton Seal for being smart, funny, and rather ace; the wonderful, inimitable Dr James Barrett for always making me feel as if I should be doing a bit better, while also being entirely ok just as I am; and Dr Sarah Murjan who, being both incredibly smart and equally kind, so often lets me have space to pontificate in her office before a gentle "I suppose there's also . . ." which is invariably the better, kinder thought that gives me pause. Lastly, I would like to thank the late Sir Terry Pratchett, whose words have given me a home when the maelstrom threatened to sweep me away and whose philosophy may just be the wisest thing yet written.

Chapter 1

Introduction

Transgender people – most commonly referred to as simply trans people – are just like cisgender[1] (non-trans) people in that the vast majority of life is spent doing the things that people do – working, studying, playing, laughing, crying, having sex, not having sex, eating buns – all the stuff of life. There are, however, a few key considerations relating to trans and it is some of these, especially to do with sexuality, which this monograph covers.

But what is *trans* when used in this context? Briefly it is an umbrella term which includes a variety of different identities – all of which are concerned with a person living all, or a part, of the time in a gender other than that to which they were assigned at birth. Within the psychiatric literatures these have previously been split into differing groups: In the as yet current World Health Organization's (WHO) International Classification of Diseases (ICD) these are *transsexualism*, in which a person wishes to live all of the time in a gender other than they were assigned at birth; *dual role transvestism*, in which a person lives in that manner for part of the time; and *fetishistic transvestism*, in which there is a sexual component to taking on the role of another gender (WHO, 1992). It is likely that *transsexualism* will be renamed *gender incongruence* in the forthcoming 2018 edition of the ICD. The more recently published *Diagnostic and Statistical Manual of Mental Disorders* (DSM-5) of the American Psychiatric Association (APA, 2013a) elides the first two categories of transsexualism and dual role transvestism for diagnostic purposes under the category *gender dysphoria*, which might also include people who identify as something other than male or female. The DSM 5 also includes the category of *transvestic fetishism*, which roughly correlates with *fetishistic transvestism* in the ICD. In the DSM, but not in the ICD, there is a requirement that there be "clinically significant distress or impairment in social, occupational, or other important areas of functioning" (APA, 2013a, p. 702). However, somewhat unusually, the diagnosis is often made without this distress in order for robust and supported trans people to access physical assistance to align their bodies with their minds (Murjan & Bouman, 2015).

There is consequently much contention around having diagnoses associated with gender role and identity, given that there are not necessarily any problems with living associated with them[2] (cf. Karasic & Drescher, 2005). Indeed, the terms *transvestite* and *transsexual* have a history of pathologisation associated with them (cf. Karasic & Drescher, 2005), and these words are only partially reclaimed by some members of the communities – in the sense that some people are happy to use them and many are not. Nonetheless, shorn of pathology, these three rough groupings – people living full time in a gender other than that assigned at birth; people living part of the time in a different gender; and people for whom the endeavour appears to have a sexual component – can be a useful heuristic under some circumstances (Barrett, 2007; Ettner, Monstrey & Eyler, 2007; Richards & Barker, 2013). Notwithstanding this, the APA (2013a) and WHO (1992) note that fetishistic stages can precede the wish to live in another gender role, which makes clear demarcation between the different categories somewhat problematic; and further Lawrence (2013) contentiously asserts that, for trans women[3] at least, it is possible that there is a sexual component to a cross gender [transsexual] identity.

Two further rough groupings of people who may fall under the trans[4] umbrella are gender neutral people – those people who identify with no gender, sometimes referred to as neutrois, agender, or gender neutral people (Richards & Barker, 2013) – and non-binary or genderqueer people – those people who have both genders simultaneously to varying degrees (or who disagree with the binary gender system) (Richards & Barker, 2013; Richards, Bouman & Barker, 2017). These groups of people are emerging communities and a burgeoning political force. Therefore, further research into any necessary or useful assistance such as hormones, surgeries, therapy, and so on for these groups will be required – which is one of the reasons the DSM-5, and likely the ICD-11 have included these gender forms in the diagnostic categories such that aid may be rendered as necessary. There is almost no research or writing on these gender forms, with the exception of Richards et al. (2016); Richards, Bouman & Barker (2017); student dissertations (Evans, 2011); and some community publications (e.g. Bornstein & Bergman, 2010; Diamond, 2011; Queen & Schimel, 1997[5]) with what little there is generally falling under the wider umbrella of studies on trans identities.[6]

Given this complexity, members of the trans communities[7] themselves generally use the overarching term adopted in this paper – *trans* – to include all of these practices and identities (Bornstein & Bergman, 2010). Because of this, in this monograph the concept of trans will be assumed to mean *living some or all of the time in a gender not assigned at birth*. Of course, this does not fully encapsulate the difficult issue of identity, especially within an existential framework (which is discussed below), and indeed, self-definition forms a key part of this phenomenological research. So, while the working definition above is included for clarity, it should not be seen as a structural or theoretical imposition of meaning on participant realities.

Similarly, sex and sexuality are complex and often ill-defined terms both within general discourse and in the grey and academic literatures. Sex, for example, might pertain to chromosomes, coitus, something like *gender*, etc. Sexuality is a little clearer with the Oxford English Dictionary defining it as "capacity for sexual feelings"; "a person's sexual orientation or preference"; and "sexual activity" (Oxford Dictionaries, 2015a); with *sexual* pertinently further defined as, "Relating to the instincts, physiological processes, and activities connected with physical attraction or intimate physical contact between individuals" (Oxford Dictionaries, 2015b). To complicate matters still further, *asexuality* – not experiencing sexual attraction (AVEN, 2017) is also often regarded as a 'sexuality' in much the same way atheism is often included within demography sheets under religion – and with all the same subtleties of degree and type that one might expect in any human practice or identity. Consequently, the definitions above are the broad working definitions used in this monograph; however, for the reasons touched upon above and detailed below, such matters are complex when considering trans people, and indeed it is this complexity which this research seeks to explore.

These complexities around both trans and sexuality, and especially their intersections, have been addressed within literatures from a positivistic tradition (such as medicine and essentialist psychology); and theoretical academic literatures (including queer theory and postmodernism), both of which sometimes appear to utilise trans people's realities for their own ends. Thus medicine has been accused of appropriating trans voices to buttress the gender dichotomy[8] (Raymond, 1979), whereas (rather ironically) queer academics have been accused of appropriating trans experience to buttress arguments *against* the gender dichotomy (Richards, Barker, Lenihan & Iantaffi, 2014; Rubin, 1998).

Where then is the counselling psychologist with a trans client to turn for information on trans experience which is free(er) from such theoretical (and so methodological) bias? Phenomenological enquiry may have an answer. Other valid methods are discussed below (as are issues with phenomenology itself), but the great strength of phenomenology is the rigorous investigation of "things as they are in themselves" (Husserl, 1970 [1900]) which would seem to be just what is needed amidst the brouhaha of enquiry into trans, both within the academy and beyond (cf. Green, 2008). Phenomenology also neatly intersects with the field of Counselling Psychology as it is a very common mode of therapeutic enquiry for counselling psychologists (Woolfe, Dryden & Strawbridge, 2003) – whose credo puts great value on the lived-experience of the client. This credo also recognises the centrality of intersubjectivity for counselling psychological practice (HCPC, 2012; Orlans & Van Scoyoc, 2009) which is something that, it may be argued, is best facilitated though a full phenomenological investigation of the clients' 'worlding' (Spinelli, 2007).

One important area of trans clients' worlding is, as we have started to touch upon above, that of sexuality. Trans people's sexuality forms much of the literatures on trans in general and indeed is one of most contentious topics within this field (Dreger, 2008). Again, phenomenology which privileges meanings – rather than a theory-driven method which seeks certain 'data' (sometimes without due regard for individual differences – cf. Clarkson, 2008; Richards, 2017b) may be a fecund mode of enquiry. Phenomenology alone, however, could risk leaving the experience of trans sexuality[9] in a vacuum. The endeavour to situate such experience within a philosophical framework therefore needs to avoid the pitfalls sketched out above in terms of theory driving research, but still needs to find some 'firm ground' from which to work without the use of 'grand narratives' (Lyotard, 1984). For this reason existentialism offers a philosophical base and hermeneutic (historically intertwined with phenomenology – van Deurzen & Adams, 2011) which may be used to tentatively investigate the phenomenology of trans sexuality, but which itself has few distorting theoretical a priori assumptions (of the 'meaning' of trans especially).

The research in this monograph therefore, is an existential-phenomenological investigation of a group of trans people's sexualities. It critically considers the literature on trans sexuality and seeks to justify the method chosen for exploring trans sexuality with particular reference to ethical considerations of this generally psychologically robust, but sometimes culturally marginalised and academically exploited, group. It then turns to the results of a study undertaken with a group of self-defining trans people and considers the theoretical context of these results within the discussion. There will necessarily be no reporting of 'answers' fixed and true for all time, but rather a series of non-generalisable themes are highlighted, which should be held lightly to be properly seen (Richards, 2011a), thus becoming part of an ongoing and hopefully fruitful dialogue within academic, clinical, and, it is to be hoped, community circles.

Lastly, as they read I hope the reader will forgive my, at times, somewhat personal use of language – of reflections about my own work, thoughts, and feelings. I feel that as a counselling psychologist it behoves me, unless there is cause otherwise (see reflexivity below), and in so far as is possible, to speak to you the reader as a person – without endeavouring to hide the fact that we are both human – and so there will be some degree of intersubjectivity between us. This will, of course, be rather limited by the medium. Indeed, as I am unable to respond to your reading except in my imagining of what that response may be, perhaps rather than actual intersubjectivity it would be better to say that I am endeavouring to respond to you as a *person*, as a reader with both your expert knowledges and our humanity available to us. I shall don my scientific tweed and passive voice as proves necessary then, but where I leave it hanging on the chair and speak to you directly I beg your forbearance as – to me at least – somewhere in all that is something important in being a counselling psychologist.

Notes

1 A cisgender person is a person who is content to remain the gender they were assigned at birth (Richards & Barker, 2013).
2 Of course this book series is entitled *Explorations in Mental Health*; however, this is not to say that gender diverse matters are mental health matters, as of course they are not. They may inflect and impact upon mental health, but are not mental health matters per se. The

inclusion of this book in the Series is to inform people when these matters do affect mental health, but should not be taken as tacit agreement that gender diversity is necessarily about mental health, as it is not; there is a very great deal more contained within this volume, as we shall see.

3 A trans woman is a person who identifies as a woman and who lives in a female role, but who was assigned male at birth. Similarly a trans man is a person who identifies as a man and who lives in a male role, but who was assigned female at birth.

4 Some people have used the term *trans★* to refer to a wide variety of trans identities with the '★' being a wildcard term from computer programming denoting a variety of possible endings, for example trans-sexual, -vestite, -gender, etc. It also includes a number of terms which don't have the strict morpheme 'trans' in them, but which nonetheless fall in the same rough category, including gender neutral and non-binary gender. Useful as it may be, it can be difficult to read (especially aloud) and, most importantly, at a recent meeting of trans community leaders we convened as part of my clinic's research for the WHO on the ICD-11 it was unanimously felt to be an exclusionary term which people not keyed into the latest developments in trans may be unaware of – and may therefore serve to marginalise people further. For this reason it is not used in this monograph.

5 Which was twenty years ahead of its time.

6 And occasionally getting wet as they are pushed out from under that umbrella when the street gets bumpy.

7 I should note here for reasons of clarity that, while I shall touch upon cross-cultural considerations below, I am referring to trans communities from high GDP Western countries.

8 The gender dichotomy is the notion that there are only two genders (male and female) which are different in kind rather than degree (Bockting, 2008).

9 Trans sexuality (the sexuality of trans people) should not be confused with *transsexuality* which is a diagnostic term pertaining to those people who live, or wish to live, permanently in a role other than that assigned at birth.

Chapter 2

Literature review

Literature search method

The following literature review started, as many literature reviews do, with an accumulation of my literature on this topic to this point in time – the contents of my bookshelves and hard drives if you will. Given my other academic work in this field, mentioned throughout this monograph and elsewhere (cf. Richards, 2017a), this seems a reasonable start to an overview of the field. I have also spoken to both academic and clinical colleagues in the field of trans and sexuality, as well as in counselling psychology, existentialism, and phenomenology who have suggested titles which I have pursued both in reference to other work and to this monograph specifically. Naturally, this has led to a snowball literature search with pertinent references being sought as papers and books have been examined.

In addition to the above, a formal literature search was carried out using search terms which seemed from a nominal perusal of the literature, and my prior work, to be pertinent to the current study. These were (in alphabetical order): Gender neutral; Non-Binary Trans; Trans★; Transgender; Transsexual; Transvestite. Additional terms which were added to these were Existentialism;[1] Phenomenology;[2] Sex; Sexuality. These terms were used in the following research databases: AMED, BNI, CINAHL, Embase, HMIC: DH–Data and Kings Fund, Medline; and PsychInfo, as well as Google Scholar and Ovid (see Tables 2.1 to 2.3 below). The term *Transsexual* alone returned a very large number of results (3077) with many erroneous responses pertaining to other matters. Thus only papers with secondary specifiers were included. Of these, several, especially those containing the terms *Trans* and *Trans★*, also returned large numbers of hits, as the search engines didn't discriminate between trans(sexual) and translator, trans-acids, trans–disciplinary, etc., giving rise to erroneous hits regarding maize, for example (Chandler, Eggleston & Dorweiler, 2000). In these cases only the first hundred hits were reviewed as the papers were ordered by relevance and after this point the relevance markedly decreased. In addition, several of the search terms will overlap, for example trans and transsexuality often returned similar results, meaning the number of hits cannot be summed.

Table 2.1 Number of returns on database search

Gender form	Additional specifier			
	Existentialism[3]	Phenomenology	Sex	Sexuality
Gender Neutral	0	3	554	59
Non-Binary	0	0	4	3
Trans	1	25	1940	151
Trans*	110	3612	137,598	8367
Transgender	1	9	1561	8
Transsexual	1	4	1216	136
Transvestite	0	11	138	15

Table 2.2 Number of returns on Google Scholar search

Gender form	Additional specifier			
	Existentialism	Phenomenology	Sex	Sexuality
Gender Neutral	3300	3790	50,900	33,400
Non-Binary	956	572	2270	2360
Trans	25,500	187,000	2,280,000	342,000
Trans*	25,700	183,000	2,310,000	338,000
Transgender	5190	6110	41,700	34,500
Transsexual	3190	3890	25,700	19,000
Transvestite	3730	3160	18,100	12,300

Table 2.3 Number of returns on Ovid search

Gender form	Additional specifier			
	Existentialism	Phenomenology	Sex	Sexuality
Gender Neutral	0	0	5	0
Non-Binary	0	0	0	0
Trans	251	3691	22,559	3363
Trans*	251	38475	784,341	62,450
Transgender	16	231	7751	4442
Transsexual	8	117	4378	1490
Transvestite	2	32	604	257

The search terms on their own did not return a sensible structure for this research and consequently the literature review incorporates all of the pertinent papers across the following sections as necessary. Naturally this starts with the history of trans people and some information on the place of trans people cross-culturally. It then turns to the rates of trans people within mainly contemporary Western populations as this is the primary demographic focus of this monograph. As one of the key foci of contemporary Western discourses of trans is the 'psy' professions, it is to this we turn next – with sexuality and gender inflecting much of the work here. This is followed by an in-depth consideration of sexuality and gender specifically; which leads on to trans people's partners, sex work, and HIV risk. Although most of these literatures concern peer-reviewed work from within the academy, community literatures will also be considered before turning finally to the specifically existential canon regarding trans and sexuality. However, it is the first of these – history and demography,[4] to which I now turn.

A history of trans people

One might assume that trans people are such a rarity that they would not trouble the day-to-day work of the counselling psychologist, however, the literature appears to suggest otherwise: Trans people in the widest sense have been found in what might reasonably be referred to as all times and all places, dating from the stone age to the present day (Feinberg, 1996; Herdt, 1996). In addition, trans people have been found in the Americas, Europe, Asia, Africa, the middle East, Polynesia, and amongst the Inuit, to name just a few peoples – although, of course, the expression and understandings of gender varies widely with time and geographical location (Coleman, Colgan & Gooren, 1992; de Cuypere, 1995; Feinberg, 1996; Gooren, 1984; 1990; HBIGDA, 2001; Herdt, 1996). Without wishing to write too much on the geographic and chronological distribution of trans people, a few examples will hopefully assist the reader in understanding the ubiquity of the distribution of trans people, but they should in no way be considered to be exhaustive.

One key example is in Northern India where the Hijra are a group of people who were assigned male at birth, but who live as 'third gender',[5] or quite often as women, and who are devotees of the Bahuchara Mata. They may carry out a variety of ceremonial purposes relating to Hindu religious practice (Kalraa & Shahb, 2013; Richards, 2017b). Hijra may gain their spiritual power through removal of their genitals and through living as women and often live in all-Hijra communities. However, as with many such identities, there are people who identify as Hijra outside of this strict definition, and some people who historically might have so identified may now be using the term *khwaaja sira* (meaning something like *eunuch* or *transvestite*, but defying strict translation into English) instead of Hijra and/or identifying within the idea of transsexualism.

Another group of people who may be considered to be trans in the wider sense are the *two-spirit* people indigenous to America. Two-spirit people may generally be birth-assigned males who take on aspects and roles of femininity, or birth-assigned females who take on aspects and roles of masculinity, but they need not take on all of the aspects or roles of the 'other' sex. In a similar way to the hijra, two-spirit people may traditionally have had a spiritual and healing role as a medicine person (in the first nation sense of the word) or as a nurse, etc., although this is by no means always the case with two-sprit people holding a variety of roles within society. There are various terms used by first nation peoples for two-spirit people such as *wíŋkte* by the Lakota, *hwame* by the Mohave, *nádleehé* by the Navajo, and *ilhamana* by the Zuni as well as several others. These terms are not exactly analogous, and indeed *ilhamana* defies direct translation into English – a point which is worth bearing in mind for readers who are rooted in a two-sex/two-gender cultural system (cf. Richards, 2016). *Two-spirit* itself is not a term which is universally accepted, as it suggests a spiritual/cultural system which does not accord with all first nation understandings and is only used as a loose umbrella term here. Indeed it is worth noting that, such is the diversity of the peoples discussed, there will be many people who identify as something outwith the terms used here.

Similar to the Hijra and the two-spirit people, the Samoan *fa'afāfine* (lit: the way of a woman) may be considered to be trans or 'third gender'; although again in a different way and within a specific cultural context which inflects basic understandings about the world. For example, Herdt (1996) suggests that, while gender liminality in Polynesia is generally accepted, it is not afforded status of a third gender within cultural praxis. The *fa'afāfine* are usually birth-assigned males who foreground traditionally feminine behaviours at certain times and are often especially engaged with their community. Within Polynesia there are also other gender groups such as the *māhū* from Hawaii and Tahiti who are birth-assigned males who have feminine gender identities and roles and are attracted to men; and the *fakaletī* of Tonga who are birth-assigned males who identify as women. In Thailand the *Kathoey* are birth-assigned males who either identify as feminine or female, and many therefore seek hormonal and surgical assistance to feminise their bodies.

Historically, the Neolithic 'goddess' Çatalhöyük evolved into Cybele, whose worship spread from Asia to Phrygia and into ancient Greece in about the 6th century BCE, where she had a uniquely trans-female priesthood (Feinberg, 1996). Unrelatedly, but only a little after this, in the fifth century BCE, Herodotus refers to the Scythians being diseased with *morbus feminarium* in what was supposed to be divine retribution. He called them *Anandrii* (Murjan & Bouman, 2015) and described them as follows:

> Their beard falls off; their genital organs atrophy; their amorous desires disappear; their voice becomes feeble; their body loses its force and energy, and at last they come to a condition where they partake of feminine costume, and assimilate to women in many of their occupations.
>
> (Beard, 1886)

In Rome in 390 BCE, laws were enacted condemning the "infamy of the manly body transformed into the feminine one" (Cantarella, 1992, p. 177), suggesting that trans practices continued at that time. And indeed they continued thereafter. Staying within Europe (although of course trans practices and identities were occurring elsewhere also) trans was frequently elided with witchcraft and condemned by the Christian church, as in the synods of the sixth and seventh centuries. For example, in the ninth century a popular guidebook dictated penance for men who cross-dressed and in the thirteenth century an inquisitor in France denounced cross gender expression (Delcourt, 1961). All of this occurred, of course alongside a great number of phenotypically female 'male' saints such as Pelagia, Margarita, Marinus, Athanasia, Eugenia, Appollinaria, and many more, as well as the (in)famous legendary pope Joan.

More recently, Feinberg (1996) reports that between 1707 and 1730 Societies for the Reformation of Manners launched attacks against "effeminate sodomites amongst the London poor" (Davis, 1975, pp. 167–168) who were then called Mollies and who congregated in Molly Houses. Feinberg reports that on one occasion in 1725 (in a striking parallel to the Stonewall riots over three hundred years later) the oppressed (trans) 'mollies' "many of them in drag met the raid with determined and violent resistance" (ibid).

In the modern era we can trace trans through a series of pinpoint examples of trans people who became known about in the wider culture from Elbe (Murjan & Bouman, 2015) to Cowell (1954) to Mahlsdorf (1992) to Jorgensen (1967) to Cossey (1992) to Bornstein (2012), Wilchins (1997), Whittle (Self & Gamble, 2000) and so to Serano (2007) and Bergman (2009) and thus to Dana International, and later Conchita, winning the Eurovision song contest, Anna Grodzka being elected as a member of the Polish parliament, and trans woman Laverne Cox on the cover of *Time* magazine.

Rates and ratios of trans people

It seems, therefore, that trans people are fairly historically and globally ubiquitous, although actual rates of trans, and transsexuality specifically, in the general population are hard to obtain. This is because many trans people do not require or seek treatment, meaning they never come to the attention of demographers. Notwithstanding this, the World Professional Association for Transgender Health (WPATH) suggests that 1:12,000 people assigned male at birth[6] are transsexual with 1:30,000 people assigned female at birth being so – giving a ratio of 1:2.5 (HBIGDA, 2001). The American Psychiatric Association put the (global) rates at 14:100,000 for people assigned male at birth and 3:100,000 for people assigned female at birth giving a ratio of 4.6:1, although they note that this varies between 6:1 and 1:1 with Japan and Poland having reversed sex ratios, and all figures likely to be rather low due to data collection methods used (APA, 2013a). In Belgium de Cuypere et al. (2007) found rates of 1:11,900 people assigned male at birth and 1:30,400 people assigned female at birth giving a ratio of 1:2.55 whereas in Singapore Tsoi (1988) found (comparatively high) rates of 1:2900 people assigned male at birth and 1:8300 people assigned female at birth giving a ratio of 1:2.86. These studies mainly concerned people approaching Gender Identity Clinics (GICs), which one might imagine would mean that the participants may be rather more committed to their trans identities, or requiring of physical change, than people drawn from other sources – and so would suggest a smaller ratio of trans to cisgender people in the general population. Indeed, in a primary care study in Scotland Wilson, Sharp & Carr (1999) found rates of: 1:7440 for people assigned male at birth 1:31,153 for people assigned female at birth with a sex ratio of 1:4.1. Using similarly good quality data, the Calderdale NHS Primary Care Trust reported that 1:5000 (0.02%) of its population were seeking some form of trans-related healthcare at a ratio of 1:4 people assigned male at birth to people assigned female at birth respectively (NHS Calderdale, 2009); using New Zealand passport holders' information Veale (2008) found (estimated) rates of 1:3639 people assigned male at birth and 1:22,714 people assigned female at birth giving a ratio of 1:6.24, although Veale suggests this sex ratio may be due to an over inclusion of people assigned female at birth in the data set which did not have a gender marked. Within the US, eminent psychologist Randi Ettner suggests that (although not necessarily identifying as transsexual or seeking services as in the examples above) some 8–10% of the US population has a degree of gender dysphoria[7] (Ettner, 1999). This implies that, far from being a niche concern, trans people are not uncommon, and indeed may be becoming more common (Reed, Rhodes, Schofield & Wylie, 2011) – or more likely, given some of the biological research on aetiology discussed below, simply more visible.

Consequently, although trans people are no more likely than the general population to have any form of psychopathology (Cole, O'Boyle, Emory & Meyer III, 1997; Colizzi, Costa & Todarello, 2014; Haraldsen & Dahl, 2000; Hill, Rozanski, Carfagnini & Willoughby, 2005; Hoshiai et al., 2010; Kersting et al., 2003; Simon, Zsolt, Fogd & Czobor, 2011), given these population numbers and distribution it is likely that some trans people will seek the services of a counselling psychologist for a variety of matters, much as the rest of the population does (Firth, 2015), but may nonetheless still require sensitivities pertaining to their life circumstances, including their sexuality.

The relation of trans people to the psy professions

Unfortunately, trans people have not been well served by psychology and psychiatry in the past (Dickinson, Cook, Playle & Hallett, 2012), especially in the time period where Western medicine took over from much religious teaching regarding morality. Prior to this, as seen above, trans expression was often prohibited by religious edict or exegesis and indeed it has been argued that much of the current medicalisation of 'paraphilias' has been as a result of the secularisation of such 'sin' into a medical discourse (Bullough & Bullough, 1977). This was driven by such works as Krafft-Ebing's (1886) *Psychopathia sexualis: Eine klinisch-forensische studie* (Sexual psychopathy: A clinical-forensic study); Ellis' (1897–1928) seven volume series *Studies in the Psychology of Sex*; and Hirschfeld's (1938) *Sexual Anomalies and Perversions* which sought to bring into a 'scientific' medical framework sexual and gender variation which had previously been considered sinful or, occasionally (and usually prior to the eighteenth century), as part of natural variation. Thus as sin moved into medicine and out of ecclesiastical delineation it became 'perversion' (Morgan & Ruszczynski, 2006), or 'paraphilia' as in the American Psychiatric Association's (APA) Diagnostic and Statistical Manual (DSM), Version 5 (APA, 2013a); and the World Health Organization's (WHO) current International Classification of Diseases (ICD) Version 10 (WHO, 1992). More recently, there have been contentions around whether there should be medical intervention into some sexuality and gender matters at all – as in the imbroglios over masturbation, 'nymphomania', and the removal of homosexuality from the DSM-III (Minton, 2002).

Historically there was little discrimination made in medical and public circles between transsexualism, same-sex attraction, and transvestitism. For example, Krafft-Ebing (1906) writes – nominally of homosexuality – "Feeling, thought, will, the whole character, in cases of the complete development of the anomaly correspond with the peculiar sexual instinct, but not with those which the individual represents anatomically and physiologically" (p. 336). Indeed, the term *transsexualismus* was introduced as late as 1923 by German sexologist Magnus Hirschfeld, and American sexologist David Oliver Caudwell introduced the term *transsexualism* in 1949 only for those wishing to change physiological sex. However, he regarded surgery as an unacceptable treatment and advocated that transsexualism should be seen as a mental disorder.

Consequently trans began being listed as a mental disorder in the ICD-8 (WHO, 1965) and the DSM-III (APA, 1980) prior to which it was not considered to be a discrete condition (cf. Meyerowitz, 2002). There has been much debate around whether it should continue to be retained within a psychiatric taxonomy given (as detailed below) there is no attendant psychopathology beyond that associated with minority stress. This change in conceptualisation has led many people to suggest that it is inappropriate to continue to diagnose trans as a mental disorder (cf. Ault & Brzuzy, 2009; Bockting & Ehrbar, 2006; Drescher, 2010; Karasic & Drescher, 2005; Lev, 2006; Meyer-Bahlburg, 2010; Winters & Ehrbar, 2010). Some people have argued, however, that trans feelings may be the cause of anxiety or distress, and so, while not in themselves psychopathological, they should be retained within the psychiatric taxonomies (APA, 2013b); others, including myself, have responded by suggesting that psychiatric taxonomies do not (and should not) generally list *causes* of anxiety and depression, but rather symptoms and syndromes (Bentall, 2003; Richards, 2007; 2015) – and that were one to list all of the potential causes of distress in human beings, the DSM and ICD would be prohibitively long. Indeed it has been questioned why it is these particular causes of distress relating to gender and sexuality (and not other matters) which have been chosen for inclusion in these taxonomies, and arguments have been made that this is a moral judgment where removal would be a "public relations disaster for psychiatry" (Spitzer cited in Kleinplatz & Moser, 2005, p. 137).

However, we might perhaps more charitably consider the bureaucratic need for some form of diagnosis for those people seeking assistance with associated distress in order to access treatment – the argument against this being that an Anxiety or Depressive Disorder alone would serve equally well, without the need for a stated cause in the diagnosis itself. Nonetheless, this argument for a bureaucratic and pragmatic need to retain the diagnoses is the one made by the American Psychiatric Association (APA, 2013b) and so the diagnoses have been retained within the new DSM-5 (APA, 2013a) as *Gender Dysphoria* (replacing *Gender Identity Disorder* in recognition that people who are dysphoric about their gender are not defacto disordered) in a new eponymous chapter all its own, and *Transvestic Disorder* which remains within the Paraphilic Disorders chapter for those people who have an erotic association with wearing clothes not normally worn by people of that birth-assigned sex. The diagnosis of *Transvestic Disorder* has specifiers relating to Fetishism and Autogynephilia[8] (although not Autoandrophilia[9]) on the basis that fetishism is likely to decrease the likelihood of a birth-assigned male developing gender dysphoria whereas autogynephilia increases that likelihood (APA, 2013a).

In contrast, it is likely that the World Health Organization will replace the current term *Transsexualism* with *Gender Incongruence* (Bouman, Richards, Whitcomb, de Vries & Kreukels, in prep) and remove it from the 'Psychiatric disorders and diseases' section and instead place it within a new section entitled; 'Conditions related to sexual and gender health' in recognition of its lack of associated psychopathology. At present, it is not envisaged that the ICD-11 will have a diagnosis pertaining to transvestitism at all as non-erotic transvestitism would be subsumed within the diagnosis of Gender Incongruence, which would be broadened to include it instead of being an updated version of Transsexualism. It is notable that both the proposed diagnosis of Gender Incongruence in the ICD and the extant diagnosis of Gender Dysphoria in the DSM contain provision for people outside the gender binary of male or female. For example, the diagnosis of Gender Dysphoria requires that one feels (among other things):[10]

4   A strong desire to be of the other gender (*or some alternative gender different from one's assigned gender*)
5   A strong desire to be treated as the other gender (*or some alternative gender different from one's assigned gender*)
6   A strong conviction that one has the typical feelings and reactions of the other gender (*or some alternative gender different from one's assigned gender*)

(APA, 2013a, p. 452)

This shift towards a more nuanced view of both gender and sexualities which eroticise transition has been encapsulated not only in the proposed and extant movement and renaming in the ICD and DSM of Gender Incongruence and Gender Dysphoria respectively, and the proposed redaction of transvestism from the ICD, but also with the addition of a clear 'Criterion B' in the DSM-5.

Criterion B is a distress or impairment criterion used in many diagnoses pertaining to sexuality in the DSM. It requires that in order for a diagnosis to be made (and so pathology to be assumed) "the fantasies, sexual urges, or behaviours [must] cause clinically significant distress or impairment in social, occupational, or other important areas of functioning" (APA, 2013a, p. 702). Thus for someone assigned male at birth to simply enjoy wearing clothes usually worn by cisgender females is no longer sufficient to merit a diagnosis.

Historically this necessity for actual dysfunction prior to diagnosis was moot as early psychoanalytic theories posited de-facto neurosis in relation to an oedipal complex, castration complexes, and 'faulty' identification with the 'opposite' sex parent (Fenichel, 1930; Segal, 1965). Other early theories included ones concerning learning and development such as the influence of parents' wish for a different sex child (Stoller, 1964) and social gender identity development (Money, Hampson & Hampson, 1957) (cf. Murjan & Bouman, 2015). While these theories have little or no evidence to support them, for some time they were considered valid and consequently both groups of people – those who have a permanent identity as another sex and those for whom the feeling is periodic – received treatment for 'perversions', 'deviance', or 'paraphilias' – sometimes because they were asked to by friends and family (Crown, 1983); sometimes because there was a problem which it was felt needed addressing by professionals (as often in the clinical literatures; Junginger, 1997); and sometimes because the person themselves felt that they were in need of treatment due to social opprobrium when, in fact, their gender presentation or sexuality was harmless (Barrett, 2007).

Treatments for atypical gender expression – whether sexually motivated or not – have included aversion 'therapy' utilising classical conditioning in which the cross-sex stimuli (such as clothing) was paired with an aversive stimuli in order to form an association and so to make the cross-sex stimuli aversive. These 'therapies' included the use of electric shocks (Marks & Gelder, 1967; Marks, Rachman & Gelder, 1965), nausea (Raymond, 1956; 1969), and foul odours (Junginger, 1997; Laws, 2001), however they had limited (or no) efficacy and are understandably controversial (Krueger & Kaplan, 2002). More recently, operant conditioning designed to positively reinforce birth-assigned sex stereotypical behaviours has been, rather unsuccessfully, used through token economies in inpatient settings (Mukaddes, 2002; Schlonski & Adams, 1997).

As these approaches have been unsuccessful, enlightened clinicians have endeavoured to help trans people though physiological interventions. One of the first reported cases of surgical interventions was Dora-R in 1921 in Germany who, under the care of Hirschfeld, underwent genital surgery between 1921 and 1930. The world wars also brought advances in plastic surgery which allowed penile construction for trans men. In 1948 Harry Benjamin, an American endocrinologist and sexologist, began treating trans women using Premarin, an equine oestrogen first formulated 1941. Testosterone was also used to treat trans males sometime after this – although the record is less clear in this regard. Harry Benjamin also formed the Harry Benjamin International Gender Dysphoria Association (now the World Professional Association for Transgender Health, WPATH) which published its first treatment guidelines in 1979, and published the seventh edition in 2011. The first standards of care for trans people in the UK were published in 2013 (RCP, 2013). Throughout the standards of care, the role of the psychologist and other mental health practitioners is emphasised, especially in terms of support and evaluation, and the role of the patient as an active participant in their own care is paramount.

Due to this change in conceptualisation of trans away from the problem-based understanding detailed above, and towards one of empowerment and diversity (BPS, 2012; Lev, forthcoming, 2017; Richards & Barker, 2013), there has also been a recent marked turn away from pathologisation discourses among those people who have such identities and practices and towards a sense of community building and support. This mirrors the community building and acceptance of homosexuality in many high per capita income nations since the late 1970s (Weeks, 1999; 2007). Such community building is often via the internet, although sometimes also through face-to-face group meetings – most commonly in large urban areas (cf. Wilchins, 1997; Bornstein & Bergman, 2010). Trans people, especially those who are part of such communities, are quite commonly aware of the debates and history regarding diagnosis and treatment which can therefore colour therapeutic relations. This is exacerbated when trans people see clinicians as a rather homogenous entity as is not uncommon both in the consulting room and the literatures. For example, the literatures quite often refer to a position taken by 'the medical model' or 'the psy disciplines' (e.g. Hines & Sanger, 2010) – thus not allowing for diversity of opinion within these disciplines, or indeed often the possibility that a person may be both trans and a clinician as I am myself.

Notwithstanding this, as we have seen, trans people have historically been ill-served by health professionals in relation to their gender and sexuality, perhaps especially within gender clinics. For example, trans people have historically had to be heterosexual in their identified gender to be thought appropriate for physical interventions – i.e. a trans man was required to be gynephilic and a trans woman androphilic (Green & Money, 1969). Similarly, trans people were expected to wear rather gender dichotomous clothing in order to be accepted – trans women were expected to wear skirts, etc., although fortunately this is no longer the case within the UK. Intersecting with this concern around the control of the lived realities of trans people's lives by clinicians is concern around the co-option of trans people's narratives and understandings of their lives by clinicians – again perhaps especially those clinicians in gender clinics who have the capacity to grant or deny access to treatments required by the trans people.

One key concern of many trans people in this area of clinical appropriation and misinterpretation of their lives, for example, is that of the concept of autogynephilia – the notion that a trans woman is erotically aroused at the thought of herself as a woman, and conversely (although with less political attention) the concept of autoandrophilia – the notion that a trans man is erotically aroused at the thought of himself as a man. Attendant to this is the use of the term *homosexual* or *non-homosexual* (relating to birth-assigned sex) to refer to the trans person's preferred sexual partners. The idea of autogynephilia was first popularised by Blanchard (1989) and was taken up by Bailey (2003) and Lawrence (2013) among others. Many people, however, vigorously disagree with the idea (e.g. Moser, 2009; Serano, 2008; 2010) as it obviates trans people's sense of gender as being to do with their felt sense of self – and not for reasons of eroticism. Similarly, the terms *homosexual* or *non-homosexual* obviate the gender of the trans person in their implicit suggestion that the birth-assigned gender is the 'true' gender. Peer-reviewed papers in major international journals such as Levine's (2014) *What is more bizarre: The transsexual or transsexual politics?* And Green's (2008) *Lighten up ladies* perhaps give some indication as to the tone of the debate. Of particular note for our purposes here, however, is that notable clinician-researchers such as Professor Ken Zucker and Professor Peggy Cohen-Kettenis (psychologists based in Canada and the Netherlands respectively) have also engaged with the construct of autogynephilia and/or 'homosexual' and 'non-homosexual' (e.g. Wallien, Zucker, Steensma & Cohen-Kettenis, 2008; Zucker et al., 2012) in their published literature, meaning that trans people who are familiar with the academic field (of which there are many; Barrett, 2007) are concerned that clinicians, both abroad and in the UK, are not respectful of their lived experiences. This naturally impacts upon clinical rapport, and further upon the constructions of trans people's understandings and realities vis-a-vis gender clinics themselves (cf. Sanger, 2010). Indeed there was a demonstration of both psychologists and trans clients when Prof Zucker spoke at the BPS Clinical Psychology Conference in 2011 (Tosh, 2011).

This wariness around clinicians by trans people is exacerbated by clinicians who concentrate on gender identity to the exclusion of other factors (indicating a lack of horizontalisation at best) and so induce marginalisation and decreased rapport in the consulting room (Benson, 2013; Scarpella, 2011), possibly further marginalising trans people in their general outlook (Kidd, Veltman, Gately, Chan & Cohen, 2011; Davy, 2010; cf. Moon, 2008). Indeed research with trans people in the UK cites fear of being discriminated against as one of the key barriers to seeking assistance – even when seeking therapy for unrelated matters (Hunt, 2014). There is also a lack of training on LGBTQ issues in general for psychotherapists (Rutherford, McIntyre, Daley & Ross, 2012) and nursing staff (among others) (Singer, 2013), with general therapists often unfamiliar with needs of trans people (Lombardi, 2001) and therapists high on trait religiosity more likely to be biased against trans people (Wilson et al., 2014). Further, therapists have been found to struggle with finding appropriate language (Langer, 2011), perhaps because sexuality and gender are complex issues which can make people uncomfortable and therefore less able to communicate effectively. On the part of the client this communication difficulty sometimes stems from fearing that they would be misunderstood (BPS, 2012), or that they may be breaking a social taboo around speaking about sexuality and how it intersects with their gender (Davies & Neal, 1996). From the clinician's perspective, there may similarly be fear around that taboo, and also concern that professional standing may be reduced through appearing ignorant (Neal & Davies, 2000). This failure to communicate effectively can sometimes lead to superficial relating in which empty, socially accepted, aphorisms are used in place of deeper interlocution and intersubjectivity (Richards, 2014b). Buber (1958) refers to this as an I-It relating rather than and I-Thou relating. I-Thou relating when applied to the work of a counselling psychologist and client in this area would mean weaving *together* an intersubjective experience relating to sexuality as it actually *is.*

Given the history above, counselling psychologists would seem especially well placed to offer a place for therapy and assistance to trans people due to the fact that counselling psychology doesn't seek to neatly encapsulate experience within a traditional (positivist) 'scientific framework' but instead "has been theoretically influenced by postmodern thinking and pluralism" (Clarke & Loewenthal, 2015, p. 281). It consequently endeavours to hold tensions – including between postmodern understandings and the wider psy field (Clarke & Loewenthal, 2015; Orlans & Van Scoyoc, 2009) – and seeks to get 'alongside' the client to explore their world phenomenologically; again something which is a step change from the impositions detailed above.

Sexuality and gender

One means of this 'getting alongside' the client is a consideration of a number of different strands of knowledge: the academic, the applied, and the community literatures – a number of different epistemologies if you will. An understanding of these can act as a means of understanding the contexts of our clients and so moving towards the more intersubjective relating, that is the *sine qua non* of counselling psychological practice (BPS, 2004). This will allow counselling psychologists to have knowledge of trans from a number of different angles such that the specific client's difficulties are able to be tentatively contextualised – naturally with the client driving such contextualisation – and good rapport established (Richards & Barker, 2013). This should allow for the counselling psychologist to see the client in a fuller sense and for the client to feel the counselling psychologist is less 'other' – and so open the possibility of co-constructing an intersubjective mode of relating. On the part of counselling psychologist this requires epoché (which, it has been argued, can never be total, Langdridge, 2007; 2014) and reflexivity regarding biases (Etherington, 2004). Consequently it is necessary to 'know (more of) what we do not know' through an engagement with the literatures which will identify possible lacuna. It will also enable consideration and expansion of what we do indeed (tentatively) hold as a valid construction which will further our understandings in order that our clients are not educating us with basic information on a topic they are engaged with (BPS, 2012).

Unfortunately for the counselling psychologist seeking simple, quality information on trans and sexuality to inform their practice, the professional literatures in this area have a tendency to be rather fraught and polemic as seen above (see also Hird, 2002a; 2002b; Wilton, 2002; Sanger, 2010; Richards & Lenihan, 2012). As we have seen, this is particularly the case where some parties suggest that transsexual people (predominately trans women) necessarily sexualise their gender (e.g. Bailey, 2003; Blanchard, 1991; Lawrence, 2013), whereas others vigorously disagree (e.g. Moser, 2009; Serano, 2008), perhaps without either group necessarily fully giving due consideration to the feelings of many trans people themselves. For this reason a small study was conducted into the sexualisation of trans people to inform and inflect the extant literature. Indeed, as mentioned in the introduction, the appropriation of trans voices has historical routes reaching back to Krafft-Ebing's (1906) medical classification of trans people and beyond. Where most work agrees, however, is that trans people's sexuality is heterogeneous, with trans people having any of the sexualities cisgender people may have (Barrett, 2007; Bockting, Benner & Coleman, 2009; Stryker, 2008). Indeed, the *Journal of Homosexuality* included a special issue in 2014 on trans people's sexuality which included (in no particular order) asexuality, threesomes, role-playing, BDSM, polyamory, stud, butch, femme, lesbian, gay, heterosexual, etc., to name only a few. Many of these papers are considered below, however some papers, such as Crawford's (2014) *Derivative plumbing: Redesigning washrooms, bodies, and trans affects in ds+r's brasserie*, need not concern us here; others, such as Bettcher (2014), are theoretical and so are included elsewhere.

One key paper in the special issue was Schilt & Windsor (2014) which included data from interviews with seventy-four trans men primarily about experiences within the workplace (Schilt, 2010) and within healthcare systems (Windsor, 2006), which was then aggregated concerning bodies and sexuality into their 2014 paper. Of course such aggregation carries with it issues of concern around whether the environment would influence the responses, and as such whether aggregation is appropriate. Notwithstanding this, of note to us here is that they suggest that their participants, instead of having a 'body', a 'gender', and a 'sexuality', have instead a "sexual habitus" which consists of Embodiment, Gender identity, Erotic ideation, Lifetime of sexual practices, and Domain of potential partners. They posit that this is a dynamic process which evolves over the lifetime. It follows therefore that as this is a dynamic process it is likely to be heterogeneous across trans people, which is similar to that which we have seen above.

Also noting a degree of heterogeneity are Doorduin & Van Berlo (2014) who used semi-structured interviews with twelve participants roughly evenly divided between trans men and trans women. As I explore below, this split of gender is not easily achieved in an objective sense, except, perhaps through participant self-identification (which is, after all a very reasonable thing to accept, provided it is identified as such in the method). Accepting this split, Doorduin & Van Berlo (2014) noted that some participants renegotiated their sexual identity as they transitioned – again in a dynamic process – with some identifying as asexual for some of the time and not at other times. Some participants reported experiences of sexual ambivalence, aversion, and sadness when considering the difference between their bodies and their identities in sexual situations. This suggested a link between sexuality/sexual expression and embodiment which Doorduin & Van Berlo (2014) report did not always abate after hormones and/or surgeries – an interesting finding which leaves open questions of the nature of sexuality and embodiment. They also noted that sexual desire changed when people had cross-sex hormones and surgeries as people re-learned which activities brought pleasure, again suggesting that sexuality may change as people undertake their transitions, but not detailing how this might come about.

Maher (2011) also investigated the experience of transition. In her study she asked three African American trans women to produce two drawings – one of a bridge connecting one place to another place, and one illustrating their experience of gender transition. This was then followed by an interview. Although only working with three participants, Mahe identified four themes from the drawings: Identity, Identity formation/evolution, Change, and Restricted affect. Six themes were also identified from the interviews being: Importance of identity, Role of family, Dislike of labels, Transphobia and societal issues, Courage to transition, and Hormones and/or surgical interventions as a part of transition. These themes reflect the findings outlined from the other papers above; of note here are the themes of evolution and change which may appear trivial in relation to trans people – but which upon closer inspection seem to have an almost fractal-like complex iteration the deeper one investigates and which have opened my thinking to the wider horizons of possibilities this implies.

Ekins (1997) also noted this idea of change, although, as his study is early, it is perhaps less nuanced than those which built upon it. Ekins used grounded theory to investigate the lives of a number of birth-assigned males engaged in "male-femaling" over seventeen years, and found that they progressed from what he termed "beginning femaling" through to "consolidating femaling" as they consolidated their female selves. This consisted of "body femaling", "erotic femaling", and "gender femaling" although as Davy (2008) notes, this was predominately in the contexts of transvestite subcultures and may not be generalisable to the trans people (female, male, or non-binary) who do not have an erotic motivation for their living or acting in a gender not of their birth-assigned sex.

Davy's own (2008) work consisted of a thematic analysis of interviews with trans people in order to investigate trans people's "bodily aesthetics" (p. 1) which Davy characterises as "a set of discourses, practices, perceptions, and experiences of embodiment" (ibid). Davy again noted heterogeneity and wielded critical theory to suggest that, unlike Ekins (1997) postulates, trans peoples' bodies can become part of their identities in a sort of feedback loop – rather than necessarily only being a reflection of that identity.

Continuing with the theme of embodied identity, Lawrence (2005) undertook a quantitative questionnaire analysis of 232 patients of one genital surgeon. Lawrence found that before genital surgery 54% of participants were predominantly attracted to women and 9% to men; after genital surgery, these figures were 25% and 34%, respectively. Of note is that 85% of participants experienced orgasm after genital surgeries. Sadly there are no papers which specifically record this data for trans men. Again this quantitative paper shows that, for those people undergoing genital surgeries at least, there is likely to be an evolving period of change involving the body, identity, and sexuality which form complex embodiment in the wider sense, and which leave open questions about the meanings of such embodiment for the people involved.

Using the qualitative method of grounded theory again, Atnas, Milton & Archer (2015) investigated the transitioning experiences of eleven trans men. Atnas, Milton & Archer (2015) created a complex and incisive model of this process which will not be reproduced here for reasons of brevity; however it is notable that key themes were Authenticity, (finding) Knowledge and information, and Making the decision to change – which again reflects the importance of time and change in the process of transition. Atnas, Milton & Archer's (2015) participants identified as bisexual (4), straight (3), gay (2), and other (2), suggesting again a degree of heterogeneity in their authentic sexual selves which is at odds with older literatures which suggest trans people are necessarily heterosexual in their identified genders (e.g. Green & Money, 1969).

Following the theme of complex embodiment after a decision to transition, Rubin (2003) investigated twenty-two trans men using the Foucauldian method of *genealogy* to consider the similarities between trans and intersex[11] people in the social world. He also used phenomenological enquiry to identify the men's lived experience and the production of their knowledge and action for themselves (of which more below). As part of this, he considered the "body-for-the-self" – being the body one is aware of being, and the "body-for-others" – which is that which others perceive and which one may be alienated from. Although Rubin (2003) does not mention this explicitly, this theory follows Husserl's (1973) differentiation between *Leib* and *Körper* as a prereflective body and the experience *of* body respectively. Of course – as Rubin (2003) notes – this notion of the body-for-others (particularly when it is markedly disjointed from one's notion of what it should be) is a key element in trans men's lives – and we might argue that of trans women and non-binary people also.

This disjoint between what one is and what one is to others was reflected in Iantaffi & Bockting's (2011) internet-based quantitative and qualitative study. Internet studies are useful, of course, in reaching many people – especially some who are hard to reach – but can sometimes lack the immediacy of face-to-face encounters. Nonetheless, they found that many trans people reference heteronormativity (and the bodily facets of this) in their relationships, but that those trans people with better mental health – as measured by a number of psychometric instruments – were less concerned by heteronormativity (and were therefore more heterogeneous). Iantaffi & Bockting (2011) suggest this puts trans people into something of a quandary as to whether to conform to societal (heteronormative) norms or to transgress these and so gain improved mental health – an important consideration in and of itself for counselling psychologists working with these client groups.

We can see then that there are a number of studies on trans gender and sexuality using a variety of methodologies which often consider the complex interplay between body, sexuality, and identity and intriguingly – in the Iantaffi & Bockting (2011) study – to the notion that an acceptance of that complexity, especially in the social sphere, may be beneficial for mental health. This complexity, of course, will also play out in trans people's intimate relationships and it is to this we turn next.

Trans people's partners

There are a number of studies which examine the experienced of trans people's intimate (usually sexual) partners. There are, however, few studies of trans people's partnerships where both parties are trans. One of these is Idso (2009), who conducted a phenomenological analysis of two couples' partnerships; in one, both parties were trans, and in the other, one person was trans and one cisgender. Although only interviewing two couples, Idso identified the following themes as being important in maintaining the relationships: Acceptance, support, identity development, and intimacy – which appears to mirror Iantaffi & Bockting (2011) in that acceptance of oneself, and acceptance by others, is a key theme. Ettner (2007) also examined partnerships where both people were trans, interviewing twenty couples (forty people) and finding that they met through gender-related services (i.e. a gender clinic waiting room) and had later sexual encounters than the general population – they also rated communication and talking as far more important than physical sexual encounters. Ettner noted that the relationships were enduring ones and that after ten years the relationships continued. Half Ettner's participants attributed this to feeling like the relationship was a "last chance", whereas half found "the abandonment of gender stereotypical role behavior exhilarating" (Ettner, 2007, p. 115) showing that abandonment of heteronormativity seems to be a key theme in several studies. This is interesting as such focus is has been placed on adherence to gender norms previously (e.g. Gelder & Marks, 1969; Raymond, 1979).

In contrast to these studies, many researchers (e.g. Sanger, 2010) seek to explain the phenomena of a cisgender person being in a relationship with a trans person without due consideration of the ethical place of the very endeavour of enquiry which positions intimacy between a trans and a cisgender person as being something requiring of research (Richards & Lenihan, 2012). This includes such studies as Freegard (2000) who examined the phenomenology of 'Living with a transvestite';[12] and Hunt & Main (1997) who considered the

"Sexual orientation *confusion*[13] among spouses of transvestites and transsexuals following disclosure of spouse's gender dysphoria" (p. 39). In general such studies found that the cisgender partners of trans people negotiate complex discourses both within themselves and with wider societies in order to maintain their sense of psychic and social integrity.

Such studies did not, however, question the role of the studies themselves in impacting that integrity though implicitly suggesting that such partnerships were worthy of study and therefore potentially outside of the norm. For this reason, there has been a call in some literature to study the everyday, including cisgender heterosexuality (Rich, 1980; Warner, 2000) – a gender and sexuality which have their own set of clinical difficulties (Farvid, 2015; Mc Geeney & Harvey, 2015; Richards & Barker, 2013) and which bear inquiry into their own realities and understandings – as well as such research being a political act of balancing against that of inquiry into trans and non-heterosexual lives. The justification for the current work in this light will, of course, be considered below.

In a similar vein Weinberg & Williams (2010) studied "Men sexually interested in transwomen[14] (MSTW)" positioning the cisgender men largely as the subject of inquiry, but not questioning fully why trans women may be interested in cisgender men, and retaining the 'exoticism' of the body of the trans women as the cultural object inscribed with meaning by the MSTW and the researchers – but not, crucially, the trans women themselves. This obviation of trans women's self meaning making (in an embodied and social sense) was reflected in Forde (2011) who, as seen above, drew on the experiences of trans people's partners' attraction to trans people to question evolutionary theory and suggested that the primary reason for intimate relationships with trans people was to offer them support (in contravention of mate selection theories of evolution regarding reproduction). Of course, this obviates many trans people's realities as people of their identified gender (e.g. Boylan, 2003; Jorgensen, 1967), and the wish of many trans people and their partners for reproductive options, assistive or otherwise (Richards & Seal, 2014; T'Sjoen, Van Caenegem & Wierckx, 2013; De Roo, Tilleman, T'Sjoen & De Sutter, 2016). Indeed, these studies of the partners of trans people struggle to capture this experience of gendered authenticity by positioning trans people as others to be cared for by their (cisgender) partners. Tompkins (2014) argued strongly against this and used an ethnographic approach analysing YouTube videos and trans conferences to research the matter. Of course there are issues with using YouTube videos in that people will present in a certain way for that medium; however this need not necessarily be at odds with their identities elsewhere. He determined that – for a cohort consisting mainly of trans men and their cisgender female partners – the partners have an erotic, affective, and romantic preference for them which is not fetishistic in nature. Tompkins therefore suggests that a sex positive trans politics (and research) will incorporate trans people as a viable sexual partner without resorting to objectification of their trans status. Of note, also, is that most the of cisgender partners in these studies were female partners of trans women who were transitioning and this is, of course, a very specific cohort as such findings may vary with different gender forms and people at different stages of their life.

Sex work and HIV risk

This objectification within some of research above can unsurprisingly also been seen in accounts of trans people's sex work. Just as much work on trans people's partners considers sexuality, but not trans people's own sexuality per se. Sadly, so too does the consideration of trans people's sex work which does not always fully explore the subjective experience and desires of the trans people themselves. Trans people undertaking sex work is more common in countries without nationalised healthcare as the funds needed for physical changes, especially genital surgeries, are beyond the amounts most people, trans or otherwise, could usually hope to afford. For this reason much of this research has been done on trans people in the US where, until recently, Medicaid did not cover trans-related treatments. As trans sex work is so common in such economic regions, rates of HIV are correspondingly high (with shared needle use adding to the issue as people address their dysphoria though narcotics); one US study, for example, put HIV at a prevalence of 2.7% in trans women and 0.5% of trans men (Habarta Wang, Mulatu & Larish, 2015). The reasons for this appear to be manifold – for example Clements, Kitano & Wilkinson (1997) found that low self esteem in trans women led to risky behaviours in sex and that in trans men there was a higher rate of risky sex (Kenagy & Hsieh, 2005). Trans women were also more likely than trans men to use protection in sex work (Kenagy & Hsieh, 2005); however Nemoto, Operario, Keatley & Villegas (2004) noted that trans women also used unprotected sex to demonstrate love and commitment just as many heteronormatively married people do. Herbst et al. (2008) found that 48.3% of trans females had casual sex; Bockting, Rosser & Coleman (2000) found that trans males had poor sex negotiating skills; and shockingly Clements-Nolle, Marx, Guzman, Ikeda & Katz (2001) found that 59% of trans males had been raped.

The disturbing figures above are not representative of the bulk of trans experiences of sexuality (Lenihan, Kainth & Dundas, 2015; Richards & Barker, 2013), however they are worth bearing in mind as they inflect some of the community discourses around sexuality even in countries with nationalised healthcare and also reflect the some of the academic literatures on this topic. This is especially the case in terms of the heteronormativly derived discourse around the hypersexualisation of trans women and the difficulties many literatures have with considering trans men as having a sexuality at all.

Community discourses

One area where counselling psychologists could be well served in their wish to get alongside their clients is through a consideration of the phenomenological literature detailed here, and also the 'grey literatures', community literatures, and biographies that form the body of work which represents trans people's experiences from a different epistemological stance to that found within much of the academy. Indeed, Milton (2014a) comments that "Counselling Psychology prides itself on its grasp of more than one narrow therapeutic literature" (p. 17) and my hope is that this brief community literature review assists with that. In particular, my intent is that it will aid in the pursuit of the ethical thread which, it is hoped, is woven throughout this work – that the respect thus paid weighs somewhat against the imposition (appropriation?) of the academy in trans people's lives and therefore inflects both practice and research. As this is an (empirical) research-based monograph, a thorough review of literature found outside the academy will not be undertaken, but for the reasons above and also as a resource for the interested reader, community literatures are included below.

The first of the early biographies by trans people tended to be 'revelations' about people's trans lives such as Lili Elbe's Man into woman. An authentic record of a change of sex: The true story of the miraculous transformation of the Danish painter Einar Wegener-Andreas Sparre (Hoyer, 1933) about the first recorded person to undergo genital reconstruction within modern western medicine; Mario Martino & Harriett's (1977) biography (one of the first about a trans man) Emergence: A transsexual autobiography; and Christine Jorgensen's (1967) A personal autobiography which made much of her being a soldier when in fact she had extremely limited military service. Jan Morris' (1974) Conundrum: From James to Jan: An extraordinary personal narrative of transsexualism also included an interesting account of her work as a Times reporter on the successful ascent of Chomolungma (Everest). Within this time period Virginia Prince's (1971) How to be a woman though male was a seminal 'how to' book for trans feminine people. These biographies and Prince's work nonetheless helped shape popular ideas about trans people as people and away from simply being grotesques or medical curiosities and are useful material for a consideration on where some contemporary discourses on trans have come from. This work continued with excellent autobiographies such as Dr Jenny Boylan's (2003) She's not there: A life in two genders and Dr Jamison Green's (2004) superb Becoming a visible man. As with many of those above, trans people have often written biographies in which their trans status was accompanied by some other notable feature such as Mark Rees' (1996). Dear sir or madam: The autobiography of a female-to-male transsexual which told of his struggle for legal recognition, and similarly Caroline Cossey's (1992) My story in which she too detailed her efforts to gain legal recognition for her gender. Also notable was Charlotte von Mahlsdorf's (1995 [1992]) Ich bin meine eigene frau which tells of her life under both the Nazis and National Socialism.

In the 1990s the rise of postmodernism brought with it some biographies and biographical work which challenged the binary orthodoxy and its limitations, some of which included recollections of activist work by the authors. These included Leslie Feinberg's (1993) ground breaking semi-autobiographical novel *Stone butch blues*; Kate Bornstein's (1994) wonderful, seminal, *Gender outlaw* and Riki Wilchins excellent (1997) *Read my lips: Sexual subversion and the end of gender*; as well as Queen & Schimel's (1997) biographical edited collection *PoMo-Sexuals*. This trend has continued with Bornstein's (2012) updated biography *A queer and pleasant danger* and Bornstein & Bergman's (2010) edited collection *Gender outlaws: The next generation*. This is not to say that all biographical writing by, or about, trans people is now postmodern or non-binary as, while referencing such concepts, work such as Will Self's investigation of masculinity *Perfidious man* (which includes biographical work on professor Stephen Whittle; Self & Gamble, 2000), and Julia Serano's (2007) *Whipping girl*, are avowedly in support of people's self identity whether within the binary or otherwise. There are, of course, many more texts we could consider here both historically and in the present day, including many from within magazines and the internet such as Janet Mock and other's increasingly visible work. Hopefully, however, these literatures will have given a snapshot of the recording of trans people's lives within contemporary Western context. They are invaluable as they detail the lives of trans people very much as they are – albeit with the usual journalistic bias and risk of an overly positive light to mitigate the problems of these oft-marginalised groups. Notwithstanding this, the vast majority of these texts are remarkably candid and non-hagiographic. As such I find that it is useful to consider them as a means of understanding and relating to trans people as they are, in addition to the usual lens of a particular philosophical or professional discourse – and for this reason a number are referred to in this monograph.

Existential literatures

We can see then that in many literatures trans people are seen as objects on which culturally inflected messages regarding heteronormativity (resisted or otherwise) are writ large. For example, Weinberg & Williams' (2010) make the assumption that trans woman's penises are ignored if their male partner is heterosexual or incorporated if he is bisexual. As stated above, despite their heterogeneity, the experience of the trans people themselves are often lost in academic studies as cultural assumptions are played out on their (embodied) selves and lives both by any cisgender participants and by the researchers – all too often without due consideration of the ethical implications of this discourse.

What of the specifically existential literature then? Unfortunately, the existential literature on sexuality in general is still sparse (Acton, 2010; Crabtree, 2009) – with the exception of Milton's oeuvre (Milton, 1997; 2005; 2007; 2014a, 2014b, 2014c; Milton & Coyle, 2003). Indeed Cohn (2014 [1997]) notes that "Sexuality has been strangely neglected" (p. 62) and Spinelli (2014) states that "Contemporary existential authors had said little on this enormous topic" (p. 22). Although it is notable that Cohn's words from his much referenced article were reproduced in Milton's (2014b) recent (and seminal) edited collection, and some of the work touched upon below in relation to homosexuality (Medina, 2008) and affirmative therapy (Langdridge, 2014) for example, are evidence of a developing field to which this research monograph hopes to add. There have also been papers within the existential tradition such as Chung (1994) and Kahr (1994) on child sexual abuse by cisgender people, but that topic is outwith the remit of this monograph which considers only consensual sexual matters and so will not be discussed further. The existential literature on trans people's sexuality specifically is almost non-existent – with only Richards (2011b; 2014a; 2014b) and, as we see below, Leighton (1999) touching on this theme to my knowledge, and then only really as part of a consideration of trans people's experiences in the wider sense.

What extant work there is on sexuality in general in the existential canon often concerns the old argument as to whether such things as sexuality and gender can be considered to be 'Givens' in the stable, fixed, existential sense, or more ephemeral (although still deeply felt) expressions of the thrown world, which have the possibility of manifold expression. For example Cohn (2014 [1997]) argues that existential sexuality does not allow such things as a fixed identity as a gay man, lesbian woman, or indeed heterosexual person because "An existential-phenomenological perspective cannot accept the imposition of such an inflexible socio-cultural grid – without any regard for interaction, history or context – or existence" (p. 66), and further that "For the existential psychotherapist, homosexuality is not a condition brought about by specific factors, but a way of being in which whatever is 'given' is most delicately intertwined with our responses" (p. 67). Houghtaling (2013) expands upon this by theorising "sexuality through an ontology of becoming that takes into account the diverse, multi-faceted nature of sexuality as a series of temporal experiences, attractions, desires, sensations, practices, and identities" (p. ii) and that "Because both the body and the self are contingent becomings that are open to instability and change, so too is sexuality" (ibid). In a similar vein Leighton (1999) argues that existential philosophy implies that trans people should expand their idea of a given gender (which Houghtaling, 2013, characterises as a 'contingent becoming'), rather than endeavouring to transition into another gender, as seen in his statement that: "I want to see[15] men who have 'felt they were women' challenging the boundaries of what it means to be a man" (p. 160). This differs from Schilt & Windsor (2014) above, who suggest that trans men's sexual habitus is an evolving part of the self which includes embodiment, but which also allows for a stable identity as a man.

To me this suggestion that gender (and perhaps especially trans gender) is not a coherent entity reads as another appropriation of trans (and implicitly non-heterosexual) lives in the service of a stance or philosophy just as we have seen above – in this case existential philosophy rather than positivist science or postmodern queer theory. This is troubling as – while these arguments may theoretically be extended to cisgender and heterosexuality also – because cis-gender and heterosexuality are culturally accepted norms the arguments do not have the effect of destabilising them in the same way; indeed, such arguments about cisgender and heterosexuality are seldom made explicit. These arguments concerning trans and non-heterosexual lives also appear to simply ignore the lived experience of many trans and non-heterosexual people who do indeed feel as if they *are* gay, or *are* of their identified (but not birth-assigned) gender. To see why such arguments are made, however, (to understand the notation of the tunes the devil is playing if you will) it is useful to consider the underlying philosophy.

This philosophy of existential sexuality is arguably often centred within Sar-tre's notions of sexuality as objectification (2003 [1943]) in which one acquires and is acquired by the Other. This notion of being acquired by the Other is effectively an inter-*objective* phenomenon which appears somewhat at odds with his later thought on the influence of social context on the 'self'. None-theless it suggests that sexuality is an effect of this process of acquisition and is not, in itself, a *given* qua any particular individual – certainly not in the sense of Being. Sartre also suggests that an attempt to consider *a* sexuality (whether gay or straight for example) is not existentially correct, as desire must be con-tingent and situated – one does not desire all people of a given sex for example. As I explore below, there are significant issues with this as the sense of having a specific identity, linked to desire, is precisely what many people do have. Indeed de Beauvoir made similar complex arguments when considering being a woman – while being a woman is contingent "One is not born but rather becomes a woman" (de Beauvoir, 1997 [1949], p. 301), to argue that many people are not, in a fundamental sense, 'a woman', seems specious and indeed de Beauvoir herself *identified* so and (tautologically) required the identity to be available in order to make the arguments she did about a certain group of people and their desires.

The other significant stream of existential thought on sexuality is Spinelli's (2013; 2014) work (which again I explore below) and which builds upon his earlier work (Spinelli, 1996), which itself is based upon Merleau-Ponty's con-sideration of sexuality in his *Phenomenology of Perception* (2002 [1945]). In this, Merleau-Ponty viewed sexuality not as a biologically driven series of acts and feelings, but as a means of necessarily intersubjective (bodily) experience which was intertwined with existence. He stated that "Even in the case of sexuality, which has nevertheless long been regarded as pre-eminently the type of bodily function, we are concerned, not with a peripheral involuntary action, but with an intentionality which follows the general flow of existence and yields to its movements" (2002 [1945], p. 181). He goes on: "In so far as a man's sexual his-tory provides a key to his life, it is because in his sexuality is projected his man-ner of being towards the world, that is, towards time and other men (sic)" (2002 [1945], p. 183). Merleau-Ponty saw sexuality as fundamentally embodied, in the sense that the body was both a real thing in the world and at the same time the meaning it had for us: "the [sexual] bodily event always has a psychic *meaning*"[16] (2002 [1945], p. 185) and "The body's role is to ensure . . . metamorphosis. It transforms ideas into things. . . . The body can symbolize existence because it realizes it and is its actuality. It sustains its dual existential action of systole and diastole" (2002 [1945], p. 190). Spinelli (2013; 2014) largely agrees noting that (embodied) beings are necessarily intersubjective through sexuality, in the sense of sexuality being an existential phenomenon, rather than being solely an act of biological reproduction. He states that "[Sexuality's] importance lies in its ability to 'awaken' each of us to our inter-relational being" (Spinelli, 2013, p. 302), in line with Pearce (2011) who describes sex as "expression of an interacting dialectical process . . . between our given and our becoming, between interiority and exteriority" (p. 238). This is similar to Clarke (2011) who comments that "In the sexual relationship the individual goes out from himself (sic) to the other in a unity of being-with-the-other" (p. 247). Presumably the authors are considering partnered sex, or solo sex with a partner in mind (as Pearce, 2011 explicitly states), but not the (perhaps less common) sexualities which do not involve partners.

In recognising sexuality as an existential and inter-subjective phenomenon a priori labelled genders and sexualities are therefore naturally drawn into question as being fixed and at risk of creating a sedimentation, and subsequent bad faith, of what is a matter of unfixed Being (e.g. Acton, 2010). For example, Spinelli states that "It becomes evident that the correlation of sexual acts with the construction of a 'sexual identity' (be it heterosexual or LGBT[17]) imposes significant restrictions and divisions upon the human experience of being sexual" (2013, p. 305). He makes the same point regarding gender stating that "the basis for the maintenance of such constructs [as male or female] is nothing more or less than *existential choice*"[18] (ibid). Rodrigues (2014) agrees stating that:

> While we cannot even imagine existence without being temporal or embodied for instance, we can perfectly imagine it, without contradiction, without sexuality, simply because sexuality belongs to the ontic, not the ontological realm.
>
> (p. 46)

However I, for one, cannot imagine *human* existence without sexuality – we would be so different as to not be the beings which we are – in this way I assert sexuality belongs to the ontological *human* realm. Du Plock, however, appears to situate his argument concerning this somewhere in the middle – with sexuality somewhere downstream of Being and associated Givens, but still with a quite fundamental flavour: "sexual orientation may originate in a pre-reflexive manner as part of an individual's fundamental project *and then*[19] become expressed via a myriad of quotidian choices" (du Plock, 2014 [1997], p. 153) which might be depicted as something like:

Existence ⇨ Essence ⇨ Fundamental project ⇨ Choices.

However Medina disagrees, arguing that "an individual may experience their sexual preference as a natural given and furthermore something that has always been and will always be fixed" (2008, p. 13) and that "self labelling, emanating from a feeling of fixedness, provides a platform upon which each individual, despite uncertainty and doubt, can meaningfully and authentically engage in the personal challenge of being here" (Medina, 2008, p. 132). Rather pragmatically with regards to what this means for clients, Hicks & Milton (2010) note that "We need to recognise that there is a difference between the hallows of academic enquiry and people's experiences 'on the street'" (p. 262).

The difficulty with these arguments concerning essence is that there is some neuronal evidence which supports the notion of fundamental brain differences for trans people. How these differences are expressed is, of course, a different matter – but that some trans people are thrown into an embodied self which is a priori trans can no longer be in doubt. For example post mortem neuronal numbers in the central subdivision of the bed nucleus of the stria terminalis in the hypothalamus (BSTc) of trans women has been shown to be in the cisgender female range (Zhou, Hofman, Gooren & Swaab, 1995; Kruijver et al., 2000; 2004) and white matter in various brain regions of trans men has been shown to be in the cisgender male range (Swaab & Garcia-Falgueras, 2008) and grey matter sexually dimorphic regions of both male and female trans adolescents have been shown to be aligned with the gender of identity rather than birth assignation (Hoekzema et al., 2015). Many other studies have similar findings in which brain regions have shown statistical similarity to the participants gender of identity, rather than birth assignation (e.g. Bao & Swaab, 2011; Chung et al., 2002; Garcia-Falgueras & Swaab, 2008; Saraswat, Weinand & Safer, 2015). These brain regions will interact with the (social) world epistemically and so existential arguments about gender and sexuality (which are unpicked further below in relation to the intersubjective relational world, Being, and existence) should hold within them the current evidence of a biological aetiology of trans for some people.

The need for the present research in the area of trans sexuality

This notion that gender and sexuality are existential phenomena has particular pertinence for trans people as their gender (and often sexuality) is not given by society at birth (indeed it may also be an existential 'Given' as discussed above) but must instead be explicitly considered such that it is both personally congruent and socially navigable. In particular, a trans person's considered gender and sexuality appear to intersect, both on a personal and a social level. As we have seen, this is often not fully captured by a literature which is too often driven by the theorisation of trans people at the expense of trans people's own voices being heard – and it is this lacuna in the literature which this research seeks to address. For the reasons stated above, the research question is not framed in a manner which drew on positivist ontology or theory, but rather is as open as possible in order to draw in as much of the phenomena as possible. It therefore consists of a simple question:

"(As a trans person) what is your sexuality?"

Notes

1 Many authors of papers returned by search engines use this to mean something like 'deeply personal' rather than the philosophical meaning used in this monograph.
2 This term often meant something like 'the way it looks to me' (e.g. Hofer, 1960) rather than the technical sense used in this monograph.
3 The single hits here are my paper: (Richards, 2011b).
4 A term often used in the literature is *epidemiology*, however as this is associated with pathology, and I am taking an explicitly non-pathologising stance here, it will not be used.
5 This is a problematic term, assuming as it does a Western binary gender system (cf. Towle & Morgan, 2006).
6 Birth assigned refers to birth-assigned sex, thus a trans woman would be a 'person assigned male at birth'. Referring to birth-assigned sex in demographics such as these obviates the potential problem of referring to differences between gender identity (who one believes one is) and gender presentation (who one presents as being) later in life. Of course the gender of identity should be used on almost all other occasions.
7 The word *dysphoria* is the antonym of *euphoria*. The term *Gender Dysphoria* is also a diagnostic term used in the DSM (APA, 2013a), which will be capitalised here to differentiate it and so aid clarity.
8 Erotic arousal at the thought of oneself as a woman.
9 Erotic arousal at the thought of oneself as a man.
10 Italics in the following quote are my own.
11 *Intersex* is a term used to refer to the condition of having physiology which does not fall neatly into categories of either male or female. The term *Diversity* or *Disorder of Sex Development (DSD)* may also be used (Richards & Barker, 2013).
12 For ethical clarity it can be useful to hypothetically transpose another fundamentally innocuous demographic which people may find offensive. Imagine the ethical conundrum of proposing to study 'living with a black person' for example.
13 Italics my own.
14 Interestingly this is usually separated as 'trans women' (as I have done here) such that trans is a specifier of a group of women – women with a trans history if you will – rather than a discrete category of humanity: Men, women, transwomen, [transmen].
15 I'm never clear why we should care what Leighton "Wants to see"? Personally, I'd like to see a bit less philosophical arrogance and pomposity.
16 Italics in the original.
17 Lesbian, Gay, Bisexual, and Transgender.
18 Italics in original.
19 Italics in original.

Chapter 3

Method

Epistemological framework

As I have illustrated above, most past research on trans has been grounded in either a positivist, or explicitly theoretically oriented, epistemological framework. It may be argued that these are entirely reasonable approaches if the desired outcome is, respectively, to obtain 'generalisable' information about trans, or to understand its place within wider theories of gender. This section will briefly set out why such frameworks were not deemed appropriate for the current research, and why an existential-phenomenological counselling psychological hermeneutic framework was employed instead.

Research on trans people utilising a positivist methodology has often been problematic in that it has attempted to explain perceived 'difference' and not the experience in its own right, devoid of such comparison; further it most usually has also not been of explicit benefit to trans people themselves (Meyerowitz, 2002). In terms of methodological difficulties, a major issue with quantitative positivist research is that it requires discrete categories prior to the research (Coolican, 1994; Langdridge & Hagger-Johnson, 2009). These categories must, of course, be derived from some a priori source, which are usually from the researcher's assumptions and/or the established literature, which, as seen above, can be contentious (e.g. Lawrence, 2005; Weyers et al., 2009; Veale, Clarke & Lomax, 2008). For example, a research design which provides a limited set of possible categories for a trans participant's sexuality (e.g. heterosexual, bisexual, homosexual) may not reflect the lived experience of the participant who defines using terms outside of this range (such as queer, kink, furry, leather, etc.).

On occasion scientists from the positivist tradition who laud quantitative approaches suggest that the alternative qualitative human sciences approach is necessarily flawed as it is open to bias and (they argue) due to having insufficiently rigorous method it is inaccurate and therefore not 'Science'. Leaving aside mitigating efforts such as reflexivity considered elsewhere, one challenge to this is that some subjects are not amenable to a quantitative research simply because some things cannot be quantified in any sense in which they remain recognisably the subject under investigation. How much (numerically) love do we have; beauty do we find; meaning can we create? How much sexuality do we have? How much (trans)gender?

Further, we can address this quantitative bias within its own terms. Quantitative scientific method, of whatever sort, strives after perfect data – perfect measurement of discrete units with no confounding variables. Good scientists recognise this as an ideal – a striving towards a perfect method which cannot be reached, but the endeavour of which is nonetheless worthwhile. Accepting that there is 'fuzz' in whatever data we examine then, the argument against the rigour in qualitative analysis becomes a matter of degree and so falls down on those terms – whether qualitative or quantitative there is fuzz in the data and an attempt to mitigate it. The nature of the matters under investigation in qualitative analysis may mean that there is more fuzz from a positivist standpoint (just as there is more meaning from a [existential] philosophical qualitative one), but this does not make it worse, simply different – as it is a means of investigating a different matter.

Qualitative approaches might then be a reasonable option for researching aspects of such things as sexuality and gender. In contrast to quantitative approaches considered above, theoretically based qualitative research on trans generally takes a position regarding whether trans is transgressive or not (e.g. Hird, 2002a, b; Wilton, 2002), and often problematically suggests that the theory is independent of the theorist (cf. van Manen, 1997; 2014). As seen above, in some research, it also sets up a false dichotomy between trans as something to be celebrated (for subverting gender norms in sexual practice, for example) or to be criticised (for failing in such radical potential). Indeed, the complex experience of participants seems to be shoehorned into such a dichotomy, with a lack of attention paid to lived experience or to the wider discourses (Barker, Richards & Bowes-Catton, 2012; Richards, Barker, Lenihan & Iantaffi, 2014). Of course, examining lived experience is valuable in and of itself as the humanising, individual, and contextual dimensions of what this group of people (this 'research cohort' in quantitative terms) *lives* is of immeasurable benefit to wider society, as well as to clinicians of a wide variety of backgrounds in assisting them to realise *who* the people they are seeing *are*.

For these reasons, it was felt to be important that this research investigates the lived experience of trans people and their sexualities with as little bias and a priori assumption as possible. Phenomenology, which is grounded in a stance of cautious inquiry and reflective epoché (Husserl, 1970 [1900]), would seem the appropriate means of addressing such a topic and indeed a number of researchers have published on trans (although not trans sexuality) using phenomenology as their mode of enquiry (e.g. Davy, 2008; Salamon, 2010), with Idso (2009) and Forde (2011) touching on trans sexuality as part of an exploration of couples' intimacy as seen above.

Some workers have recognised, however, that the 'rich description' obtained through phenomenology often lacks a philosophical location and, as such, does not necessarily reflect the human contexts in which it is produced (Gillespie &

Cornish, 2009; Langdridge, 2013). A viable compromise may lie in an interpretative and – to some extent – context-aware analysis (rather than simply descriptive analysis; Silverman, 1984), which can remain embedded within the meanings which are produced by participants. Indeed regarding counselling work, Milton (2014c) defines affirmative practice as being "context aware" (p. 6) which points to an ethical basis for such a stance. Such an approach follows existential thinkers such as Sartre and de Beauvoir in attempting to identify the authentic themes in a person's accounts through interrogating them and being aware of the meanings that those people may be drawing upon in the world around them – since we are born into "an already meaningful world which reflects to me meanings which I have not put into it" (Sartre, 2003 [1943], p. 531). For these reasons, a philosophically grounded double hermeneutic[1] of description,[2] followed by 'suspicion'[3] (which Langdridge, 2014 describes as "the use of an external framework to uncover further layers of meaning" p. 163) may be usefully applied in analysing such material (Ricoeur, 1970). In this case, existential theory may be employed as the hermeneutic of suspicion, as its respectful grounding in human being-in-the-world-with-others (Heidegger, 2008 [1962]); allowance of heterogeneity; and freedom, choice, and responsibility (Sartre, 2003 [1943]) seem most appropriate to the material of trans people's sexuality (Richards, 2011b). Note that this does not mean the imposition of 'expert knowledge' onto the phenomena. Rather it is a cautious awareness of the possible contexts of the phenomena – which requires the rigorous application of method and reflexivity examined in the section on reflexivity below.

Additionally, phenomenology alone does not necessarily render *pragmatically* useful information. Given that trans peoples' experiences have been used to further researchers' ends and to their benefit, possibly at the expense of the participants and communities (Richards, Barker, Lenihan & Iantaffi, 2014), it seems reasonable to situate the information so elicited within a critical counselling psychological framework (BPS, 2004; Woolfe, Dryden & Strawbridge, 2003) such that the voices of the participants may be utilised to the definite pragmatic end of informing counselling psychological practice. For this reason also, the common and generally useful method of Interpretive Phenomenological Analysis (Smith, 2008) was not used as it does not explicitly utilise a *double* hermeneutic (in which a hermeneutic is specifically informed by a particular philosophy), and does not engage with the political-philosophical aspects in the way a method such as Langdridge's (2007) Critical Narrative Analysis (CNA) does, although the use of *narratives* rather than themes is restrictive here. Grounded Theory (Glaser & Strauss, 1967) similarly, while being especially careful to be 'true' to the participants' data – and eschewing the use of narrative specifically – does not explicitly situate that data within a philosophical, pragmatic, or social context. Consequently the method chosen of phenomenology using a double hermeneutic endeavoured to fulfil each of these requirements – the specifics of which, and degree to which it was successful, are discussed below.

Design

The design was intended to elicit useful information from the participants in a manner which was as comfortable as possible within the pragmatic bounds and ethical opportunities available. This involved collecting data from a group of self-defining trans people by means of visual methodology which involved the creation of models depicting participants' sexualities in LEGO® (cf. Gauntlett, 2007) and which, in turn, formed the basis of subsequent explanation and discussion by the participants. This was transcribed, checked by the participants, and then analysed by the researcher. This design drew on van Manen's (1997) suggestions for human sciences research, and utilised the double hermeneutic detailed in the analytic method section below (Langdridge, 2013, after Ricoeur, 1970). Van Manen (1997, pp. 30–31) makes a series of suggestions for human sciences research which have been adapted for this research in light of his specific focus on pedagogy rather than trans sexuality. Note that van Manen does not prescribe that these suggestions need be followed in this specific order nor that they need all be explicit and mechanistic. For clarity, however, they are discussed explicitly and separately here:

1   Turning to a phenomenon which seriously interests us and commits us to the world:

   Those having read my previous work will be familiar with my interest and commitment here. Briefly, the phenomenon of trans sexuality is one of great import in my work within two NHS gender clinics, as it forms a key element of my clinical practice. I also have a keen interest and engagement in research, policy, and practice in this area, for example I have undertaken research for the World Health Organization concerned with the revision of the diagnosis of Transsexualism in the forthcoming ICD-11, I represent the British Psychological Society at the NHS Clinical Reference Group for Gender Identity Services, and I am recognised as a Specialist in the Field of Gender Dysphoria by HM Courts and Tribunals Service.

2   Investigating experience as we[4] live it rather than as we conceptualise it:

   As detailed above, the epistemological grounding, and use of phenomenology without (as far as possible) an a priori theoretical bias, has informed this research throughout. In my clinical and academic work in this area I have also endeavoured to be aware of the cultural milieu surrounding myself and my participants (and which may appear 'ready-made', de Beauvoir, 1986 [1947]) by, for example, analysing media texts and popular cultural depictions.

3   Reflecting on the essential themes which characterise the phenomenon:

   Van Manan's use of the word *essential* is problematic here as it might imply an 'essentialist' philosophical discourse with specifically delimited knowledges.

Instead this research seeks to be reflective of the concerns of the participants. Further, the use of phenomenology, and the process of analysis, is intended to establish some such themes (although no 'Truth' is true for all times and places), as well as contextualising those themes to situate them in a wider manner within both the participant's discourses and wider discourses.

4   Describing through the art of writing and rewriting:

The double hermeneutic was applied throughout the process of transcription and through identification of themes within the texts after transcription by a process of marginal notation. As this research was written, a further process of refining the identified themes took place.

5   Maintaining a strong and oriented phenomenological-existential and counselling psychological relation to the phenomenon:

Van Manen's word *pedagogical* has been replaced with *phenomenological-existential and counselling psychological* here, as these are the concerns of this work. The strength of the orientation has been maintained through a rigorous philosophical stance towards the epistemological framework, the design of the research, and the analysis, particularly through an iterative process of engaging with the literature while undertaking the research.

6   Balancing research context by considering parts and whole.

This was addressed through the use of a method which includes a 'double hermeneutic' of description and of 'suspicion' (Langdridge, 2007; Ricoeur, 1970) to capture both the parts in the participants' contributions, and also the broader context, through the use of a hermeneutic of suspicion as outlined in the analytic method below. In addition, the context of the research itself, for example the previous co-option of trans voices, has informed the design.

The use of visual methodologies and the use of a group

Visual methodologies are particularly valuable in phenomenological research because they enable participants to provide accounts which differ from the standard scripts which are readily available through cultural and sub-cultural discourse, and in this way they may be closer to their lived experience (Bowes-Catton, Barker & Richards, 2011). A common visual method is to use photographs and indeed Davidmann (2014) has used this approach with trans people specifically, although this was a more of an artistic project with no epistemology underlying the analysis, no formal ethical approval stated, etc. Social scientists have used photography within a formal framework however, with the usual method being to ask participants to bring photographs to speak to (Harper, 2002) and indeed this has also been used with trans people specifically in the past (Davy, 2008). Photographs, however, can be a very identifiable method which can cause ethical issues as some trans people may consent to having photos published as part of research and then regret having done so as their lives move on. One way around this, as in Davy (2008), is not to publish the photos, however this too has difficulties in that the reader is then not privy to the photos the participants are speaking to. The additional problem of participants bringing photos to the researcher is that it allows for participants to prepare their responses beforehand. This was explicitly not the aim of the method for this research where it is intended that the item the participants create to speak to is constructed at the time so as to avoid accreted or prepared scripts.

Of the possible materials for such construction, LEGO® then was chosen because it does not require artistic ability, is playful, and is likely to be familiar to participants (Gauntlett, 2007) and will therefore be a comfortable form of medium for anyone who may be concerned about their artistic ability (Reavey, 2011). Indeed, such methods have been employed previously with sexually diverse groups with much success (Barker, Richards & Bowes-Catton, 2012). There are limitations to this medium in that it is pre-formed and not as fluid as a material such as plasticine – and may therefore limit possible representations. However, participants in Barker, Richards & Bowes-Catton (2012) reported that having some structure pre-formed was useful in acting as a jumping off point for their models.

Similarly, group discussion following individual explanations of the models, rather than simply individual interviews or questionnaires, was employed because this has been viewed as particularly appropriate for research with people from communities who are positioned outside of the mainstream (Basch, 1987) – as many trans people are. In contrast to individual interviews which can also elicit very rich data, group discussions are also appropriate for "exploratory research in areas where little is known" (Frith, 2000, p. 291), which is certainly the case with trans people's sexuality. Myers (1998) suggests that groups are useful for assessing opinions, attitudes, and experiences concerning a specific issue or context and the use of a group for trans people's sexuality would seem to fit this closely. Another benefit of the group discussion is that it has the potential to generate perspectives which may not have been captured in each participant's individual rich descriptions. This follows Langdridge's (2007) group methodology and previous research in the area such as Iantaffi & Bockting (2011). Perhaps for this reason groups have often been used in counselling research more widely (e.g. Carew, 2009; Widdowson, 2012).

Trans participants are likely to already know one another, as there are small numbers of out trans people who will be willing to participate in any given location. Consequently, one potential drawback of using such a group is that people may feel pressure to conform to a group norm (Fiske & Taylor, 1991; Parsons & Greenwood, 2000; Stewart & Shamdasani, 1990) meaning that individual meanings may not be elicited in deference to the meanings of the wider group. Conversely, in some group settings people can feel supported to communicate due to being a part of a group in ways which they would feel uncomfortable about were they the sole focus of enquiry. Indeed, past research on sexuality suggests that prior knowledge within a group is often positive because participants support, and gently challenge, each other based on shared knowledge, which is a useful dynamic (Kitzinger, 1994). Further, interaction between participants – whether they know one another or not – is a recognised advantage of groups over individual interviews (Merton, Fiske & Kendall, 1990) as participants can react to one another and build upon other people's contributions (Stewart & Shamdasani, 1990), as well as induce memories for other participants (McParland & Flowers, 2012). Such advantages also allow 'naturally occurring' phenomena to arise between participants, which may not otherwise occur (Kitzinger, 1994).

Notwithstanding the above, to address possible conformity bias it was made clear in the information sheet given to participants and during the session that:

> "It is important that everyone's views are respected and allowed – even if they are not agreed with by other group members. No one will say what your model means except you – neither the researcher nor the group members."

In addition, possible conformity was addressed by the use of visual methodologies, which encourages acceptance of multiple viewpoints and experiences in the same way that multiple artworks can be very different but equally beautiful (Bowes-Catton, Barker & Richards, 2011; Barker, Richards & Bowes-Catton, 2012; Reavey, 2011; Reavey & Johnson, 2008). Of course, these measures may not have been completely efficacious in ameliorating group conformity bias and it is hoped that the benefits of using a group detailed above outweigh the potential difficulties of bias.

Aside from bias, one of the difficulties with using groups can be that it makes transcribing more difficult especially if participants speak over one another (Wilkinson, 2008). This was addressed through extremely careful transcription and repeated listening to any unclear phrases. Fortunately the participants in the current study were clear and courteous in their turn-taking, which aided matters greatly.

I adhered to the guidance which indicates that between four and eleven participants are a useful number for ensuring both free discussion and a sense of safety amongst the participants (c.f. Kitzinger, 1994; Morgan, 1997). The participants were homogenous in respect to their trans status (as recommended by Basch, 1987), however, Kitzinger (1994) has also found that some degree of heterogeneity is useful for participant dialogue so homogeneity was not imposed beyond this. Indeed, participants were encouraged, both on the information sheet and in the group, to respect one another's views in order that divergence was not suppressed. For this reason, as in other studies of trans people's experience (e.g. Levitt & Ippolito, 2014), trans men, women, and non-binary people were able to be recruited as it is the experience of sexuality as a trans person which is under investigation. Further, as seen above, when researching with trans participants, defining the boundaries a priori between what constitutes men and women can understandably lead to difficulties – both with rapport and in terms of analysis – and so this was not undertaken.

Analytic method

The transcript of the participants' explanations of their models and subsequent discussion was analysed within the epistemological framework of phenomenology and the double hermeneutic described above. This involved reading and rereading with a deep engagement with the text as presented, and continual (rather than simply a priori) researcher reflexivity. On each occasion the transcript was engaged with two passes were taken and marginal notions of emerging themes were made. Each pass employed a hermeneutic of description and then a hermeneutic of 'suspicion', first to the data of individuals within the group, and then to the data from the group as a whole. Existential and phenomenological literature informed the hermeneutic of suspicion, as did understandings from the discipline of counselling psychology. This was inflected by engagement with dominant cultural meanings elicited from both the literature review and the author's other work on mainstream representations of trans people. Of course, this 'inflection' does not in any sense mean assumed prior knowledge about the participant's world views – rather that some tentative contexts and situations for the researcher's understanding had been accessed beforehand. These contexts and situations were intended, therefore, to create a situated not-knowing rather than as a means for the proof or disproof of a priori assumptions.

The double hermeneutic used is in line with Langdridge's Critical Narrative Analysis (2007) after Ricoeur (1970). However, in a departure from Langdridge (2007), but in line with van Manen (1997; 2014), the hermeneutic involved the identification of themes rather than narratives. Langdridge (2007) as well as Plummer (1995) identify the use of narratives in the 'sexual stories' of certain groups, however, the current design is specifically intended not to elicit stories as it aims to circumnavigate certain narratives (such as those which are perpetuated about trans experience). Therefore, it seems apposite to identify *themes* in line with Interpretative Phenomenological Analysis (Smith, 2008) or Grounded Theory (Glaser & Strauss, 1967).

This identification of themes further involves contextualisation, as stated above. To this end I have naturally utilised the existential literature as the primary lens for the hermeneutic of 'suspicion' situated within the wider contexts of counselling psychological understandings relating to intersubjectivity and phenomenology (i.e. Woolfe, Dryden & Strawbridge, 2003) and the field of trans studies which seeks to document and explore trans people's experience (i.e. Stryker & Whittle, 2006). With regard to the existential elements being considered, which will naturally be reviewed in full in the analysis below, I have drawn upon van Manen's (2014) notions of the 'existentials' of relationality, corporeality, spatiality, temporality as well as materiality, death and dying, language, and mood. Van Manen (2014) characterises them thus: "Existentials are helpful universal 'themes' to explore meaning aspects of our lifeworld, and of the particular phenomena that we may be studying" (p. 303). Although in his 2014 work, as in his 1997 work referred to above, he is at pains to note that in examining these facets of the ontic and the ontological it is unnecessary to consider all of these existentials in a mechanistic manner in relation to each utterance of a participant – but rather to hold them in mind during the analysis. Consequently this was the method chosen for this study, especially (linked to wider existential theory) in the second pass hermeneutic of suspicion.

It is important to note, however, that, unlike Maher (2011) it was not the models themselves that were subject to analysis by the researcher. Rather it was the participant descriptions of their own models, along with subsequent group discussion, which were analysed. This is vital, as imposing meanings on somebody else's creation is not appropriate within phenomenological analysis and could also be experienced negatively by participants. Indeed imposing meanings ignores the difficulties with shared (sub)cultural (indeed personal) understandings of what the 'red brick on the top left' generally means as there is, of course, no general meaning for it. It must necessarily be the participant's own meaning (which was the very reason for using visual methods in this research) which obviates any attempt to analyse the red brick's meaning directly by the researcher. Words, however, necessarily have *some* sort of shared cultural meaning as they are intended for communication – albeit that there is no necessarily concrete connection between intent and meaning when a given word or (with exponentially more complexity) a phrase is used. In this latter case phenomenology *seeks* meaning – but that hunt is at least not seen as a fool's errand! (I hope . . .) Consequently, images of the models are included in the analysis below in order to clarify what participants are describing rather than to aid the clarity of the analysis itself.

Reflexivity

This study utilises a phenomenological mode of enquiry (Husserl 1970 [1900])), however, it does not endeavour the complete bracketing of the researcher's position. This is because, while bracketing to the degree to which it is possible is most important; in line with Langdridge (2007) I take the view that it is impossible to have complete epoché as something of the researcher always leaks through. Indeed it seems the utmost hubris to assert that I am so self-aware as to be able to know and contain my influences – and not only that but to have no hidden areas of influence on the analysis of which I am unaware (Luft & Ingham, 1955). Consequently, the scientific rigour of the endeavour is effected through reflexivity (Etherington, 2004) and a rigorous engagement with the process of enquiry. Such reflexivity involves both personal reflection by the researcher on assumptions brought to the work, and awareness of the socio-political situation in relation to the topic of enquiry. This engagement of reflexivity, and with the phenomena of the participants, is iterative, in that both are returned to again and again – always endeavouring to ensure that the participant's voices shine through and that such of the researcher as is visible is so as a matter of decision, or a matter of clear necessity. Of course, this process too will be incomplete and so the research should be read as a conversation, with the reader taking a critical eye to the matters above (Richards, 2011a).

With specific regards to my own reflexivity about the topic under consideration, my approach is grounded by my personal interest in the field and my current career as the Senior Specialist Psychology Associate at an NHS Gender Clinic and Clinical Research Fellow at another, as well as being something of an academic in this area. It is for this reason that whenever necessary I have indicated my own published work in this monograph such that I am open to the reader evaluating my published position on the topics under discussion. Of course having such an engagement with the field might lead to 'experience assumptions' in which my prior experience inflects the work. To some extent this is precisely what is called for in the methodology used as, in line with Langdridge's (2007) CNA, contextual awareness is a requirement of the design.

Nonetheless it is, of course, imperative that the phenomena given by the participants is viewed with a 'fresh eye' to avoid undue bias in the elicitation and analysis. In supervision and elsewhere I consequently spent considerable time thinking about how to stand aside from what I have learned before as a student, as a clinician, and as an author – and so to be genuinely curious about the experiences (and indeed such continued curiosity seems to be eudemonic for me). I sought to recognise my dissatisfaction with the extant literatures which seem to be incomplete in exploring trans people's sexualities. In recognising that lacuna and endeavouring to consider how what the participants have to say might fill it – as well as contextualising participant experiences within what discourses and literature there are – I hoped to come to the information provided by these participants in a fresh and open manner. For instance, I was aware of my assumptions being overturned when I came across a contraindication to a previous assumption I had about the use of identity labels being primarily for personal rather than political ends – which proved not to be the case. Further, I am aware that over the course of writing this monograph my thinking has changed, not so much as an epiphany, but rather than a process of slow evolution which I have no doubt will continue – leading not so much towards some definite end, but rather as a part – perhaps the heart – of being (if the reader will allow me my hubris) something of a scholar and, more importantly, a person engaged with the world.

In addition (obviously), like my participants I too have a gender and sexuality.[5] I have discussed the intersections of these with my clinical and academic work both in supervision and individual personal therapy, including specific reflection in relation to this research. Such explorations enable me to approach the data in a manner that is reflexively aware "of my own thoughts, feelings, culture, environment and social and personal history" (Etherington, 2004, p. 32).

It is sometimes argued that researchers should be explicit about their own identity and history when writing up qualitative research.[6] There are, however, significant issues with including such reflexivity in academic environments and publications (cf. Richards, 2015). Participants are, of course, generally anonymised and therefore (to some extent) protected in what they have contributed to the research, however, this protection is necessarily not extended to the researcher, whose explicit reflexivity becomes a matter of public record upon publication (Etherington, 2004) – which will include, of course, a thesis lodged within a learned institution, or a monograph such as this. Thus the researcher is forced into taking a public (political) position about their own identity.

Researchers, and indeed people more broadly, who fit societally normative categories (i.e. heterosexual and cisgender people) are still far more able to be easily explicit about these than those whose identities and practices remain marginalised and stigmatised. For the heteronormative cisgender person investigating trans sexuality, for example, 'reflexivity' is often simply a matter of disavowing direct association with the matter under consideration – giving a shrugged *mea culpa* if you will (cf. Smith, 2013) – which at once excoriates and exonerates in that it suggests that there will inevitably be faults due to that personal distance from the subject, but that the heteronormative cisgender researcher cannot be to blame as they will inevitably incur these faults due to their (different, normative) identity. This done they may then continue with the business at hand content that they have 'Done Reflexivity'. (And conversely heterosexual cisgender researchers of good intent may be decried for not being able to understand, when in fact they can.) This then puts reflexivity in an explicitly political position as an undertaking – and a political position which highlights a heteronormative bias to the method.

In contrast, non-heterosexual people and trans people (who may also be non-heterosexual of course) are placed in a different position in that they risk being accused of (and indeed enacting) bias from within the groups under consideration. The difficulty is that the *mea culpa* defence seems less open to these groups – perhaps because trans isn't a norm from which to operate, but is often seen as a Minority[7] or Other which is requiring of explanation, or indeed excuse (Hall, 1995; Shepherd & Sjoberg, 2012). Indeed, as Barker (2006) asserts, people from outside normative categories risk telling 'confessional' stories, as they are frequently called upon to 'explain' themselves in a way that others are not. Public (as opposed to private) reflexivity is consequently a rather different thing for these groups with an expectation for explicit reflexivity by publishers also potentially falling foul of the Single Equality Act 2010 (HMSO, 2010) in the UK on the grounds that there is a biased material difference in favour of heterosexual cisgender people.

For both heteronormative cisgender and non-heteronormative trans researchers who are also clinicians such as counselling psychologists, there is also the risk that if clients access published reflexivity that could adversely affect the therapeutic alliance before it can be established. This would mean that for those clinicians who practice in modalities which require a *tabula rasa* such as psychoanalysis, research would effectively be precluded, and clinicians practicing from other modalities would risk their therapeutic alliance and clinical practice with each publication. This is perhaps even more the case the further a researcher moves from normativity – if a researcher wished to investigate infantilism,[8] for example, it could pose grave difficulties for them to be explicitly reflexive about their own practice within the research. This would leave the academy in an uncomfortably discriminatory position where only heteronormative cisgender people would be able to carry out research as only they could be generally able to be open about their gender and sexuality – although again here I am skating over the bias heteronormative cisgender people may face from queer communities if they are open about their heteronormative cisgender status. This means that explicit reflexivity is not a politically neutral endeavour and that there is therefore an argument that researchers, whether normative or not, should be extremely cautious about explicit published reflexivity as otherwise only those people whose personal and economic situations allow them (such as those within private practice in niche communities and those senior academics protected by tenure) will be able to be explicitly reflexive and therefore able to undertake research.

Consequently, in the current research researcher reflexivity was undertaken throughout the process, including "examining personal . . . reactions" (Finlay & Gough, 2003, p. 16), but has not always been made explicit in written form (cf. Richards, 2017b). I have obtained affidavits from my clinical supervisors as to the veracity of the claim that explicit reflexivity regarding this research has been undertaken. Of course, this does not allow the reader to consider the interpretations of the researcher given below. But given the difficulties outlined above, and given that this method of reflexivity meant it was not necessary to consider the (potentially opprobrious) opinions of clients or fellow academics during the process – and indeed utilised a method which required an ongoing supported process with other professionals, it may be the least worst option. Indeed because of this it may have actually increased the degree of real reflexivity which was undertaken and so, hopefully gives the best outcome, on balance, in terms of the validity of the research.

Ethical, moral, and legal considerations

My personal position regarding the ethics of research has continued to develop and has been discussed within supervision (Langdridge, 2007), as outlined in the section on reflexivity above. I am aware that I have a broadly positive view of trans people and so am keen to avoid further marginalising this often marginalised group (McNeil, Bailey, Ellis, Morton & Regan, 2012). Additionally, I am determined not to co-opt trans voices, as has happened too often in previous research (Richards, Barker, Lenihan & Iantaffi, 2014) – for example see Forde (2011), who utilised trans people's intimate partnerships to question evolutionary theory. I am also mindful that I am a clinician who is paid to see trans people in a professional capacity, which means that the necessity of maintaining rapport with my clients must be balanced against the aim of revealing some, albeit tentative, findings from the research. I am cautiously hopeful that the design will enable this as it precludes current or former clients from taking part.

As stated above, trans people are no more psychologically vulnerable than cisgender people (Cole, O'Boyle, Emory & Meyer III, 1997; Haraldsen & Dahl, 2000; Hill, Rozanski, Carfagnini & Willoughby, 2005; Hoshiai et al., 2010; Kersting et al., 2003; Robles et al., 2016; Simon, Zsolt, Fogd & Czobor, 2011) perhaps because, while the process of transition can be trying for some, this is not necessarily so, and indeed the process of 'becoming oneself' can involve a range of strengths and satisfactions. Trans people are, however, potentially more open to exploitation and attack (Lombardi, Wilchins, Priesing & Malouf, 2001), which could lead to anxiety and depression. Therefore ethical considerations in this study centre around ensuring that participants are not exploited, especially regarding a matter as intimate as sexuality – instead of protecting them from psychological consequences in a way which would differ to the rest of the general public. Nonetheless it was made explicit on the consent forms and debrief sheets that if anyone found the research difficult they could seek reassurance from myself as a researcher and/or approach their primary care physician, the Samaritans, or various other organisations listed on the forms given to the participants. It was also explained in detail to the participants how the data would be used such that they were reassured that the process would not be exploitative, and would potentially be of some gain for trans people in general.

In addition, in order to assist with the ethical issues of the co-option of trans voices, the design includes the opportunity for participants (but not the researcher) to review and edit the transcripts – although none elected to do so. Obviously there is a risk that useful data may be inconveniently redacted by the participants as participant and researcher understandings may differ. However, for the reasons outlined above I believe it is imperative that academic considerations do not trump ethical issues, even inadvertently, and so any 'interesting' data lost in this manner is an acceptable loss when balanced against such ethical considerations. For this reason also, the research will be 'given back' to the relevant communities through presenting it in an accessible format at community events and in community literatures (Hagger-Johnson, Hegarty, Barker & Richards, 2013).

One issue of particular concern is the identification of trans individuals as trans, given that this would constitute dissemination of Protected Information under the Gender Recognition Act 2004 (HMSO, 2004). This was addressed through meticulous anonymisation of participant identification. Under the Act trans people are, of course, allowed to disclose their trans status themselves and so disclosure within the group settings were legal given that membership of the groups was predicated upon people identifying themselves as trans.

The study conformed to all the British Psychological Society (BPS) guidelines on the ethical treatment of participants (BPS, 2009; 2010) and the relevant University ethical guidelines and was approved by the Ethics Committee overseeing doctoral research projects. Of note is that the study design required no deception. Participants were fully informed about the nature of the study prior to taking part, and their consent elicited utilising consent forms signed by participant and researcher. All participant details were fully anonymised and stored securely in encrypted form. In addition, a criterion of the consent form was that participants agree not to discuss other participants, or their contributions, outside of the group. Finally, participants were reminded that they could withdraw at any time from the research. This last was potentially problematic as until publication it would be possible for participants to withdraw. In future research of this type a time-limit for withdrawal, perhaps of one month after the data collection, is recommended.

Recruitment and procedure

The procedure was originally piloted with four trans people and then adapted (see below). In the final research, data were collected from a group of eleven trans people who were recruited through advertising a workshop at the BiCon convention in 2013. The advertisement was simply a slot in the programme entitled *Trans Sexualities* and an Information Sheet was made available beforehand.

BiCon is an annual community event originally connected directly with bisexuality, but which now creates an open space for people from a variety of sexual and gender backgrounds aside from bisexuality, as can be seen from the participant demographics, the analysis below, and Barker, Bowes-Catton, Iantaffi, Cassidy & Brewer (2008). The group was, of necessity, a convenience sample. Other options such as a specific call and arranged group might have been used; the use of a convenience sample is common in sexuality and gender work where participants are hard to reach (Barker, Richards & Bowes-Catton, 2012). The convenience sample, however, naturally carries with it difficulties in that the context the sample is drawn from may influence the nature of the participants. It is hoped that the national reach of BiCon mitigated this to some degree and the heterogeneity of the participants reflected this (see *Participants* below). Indeed all sampling methods bring with them bias – with internet requests for participants reaching people from specific groups who are necessarily computer literate, for example. It was made clear on contact, and on the consent form, that the participants must be over the age of majority (18 years of age), out about being trans, could not be current or past clients of the researcher, and could not be in an intimate relationship with another group member.

Participants were consented, in line with the *BPS code of ethics and conduct* (2010). They were advised that they may withdraw at any time with no penalty and asked for a pseudonym and basic demographic information which, with the exception of age bands, consisted of open fields in an attempt to capture the nuance of the participant's identities. The participants were then asked to create a model of their sexuality using LEGO® using the phrase "Please model your sexuality. Thank you." They would have been able to clarify what was meant by sexuality, however none did. All understood that they should not collaborate with one another; however some would occasionally pass a specific piece if it was out of reach and it was requested. In terms of the range of pieces available, there were several thousand of a wide variety of different shapes and types, with many multiples of each so as not to constrain the participants in their choice.

The participants had approximately twenty minutes to make the models, which occurred largely in silence, with the exception of a few requests for pieces to be passed as mentioned above, after which they were asked to describe their model, and what it represented, to the group. The accounts were audio recorded, as was the subsequent group discussion of the themes which emerged during the descriptions. The models were also photographed. The participants were finally debriefed and thanked.

The recording was then transcribed and emailed to those participants who elected to give the researcher their email address in order to check the veracity of the transcription. There were no changes at this stage. Following transcription, the data were subject to a hermeneutic analysis and written up.

Consequently the procedure may be summarised as:

- Eleven participants who self-identify as trans recruited (information given, consented, etc.).
- Introduction to the research provided by researcher. Potential to explore understandings of 'sexuality' if participants were unclear about what this meant (none were).
- Demographics recorded.
- Participants chose their own pseudonyms.
- Each participant made a model of their sexuality and then described it.
- The whole group then discussed trans sexuality using the models as a 'jumping off point'.
- Models were photographed, explanations and discussions were recorded.
- Participants were debriefed.
- Transcripts were sent to participants to adapt as necessary within a two-week time limit (none elected to).
- Transcripts were subjected the hermeneutic analysis detailed below.
- Themes were written up in the context of published work.
- Writing adapted for non-academic audiences and disseminated.

Adaptation after pilot study

The above design and associated considerations were originally piloted with a group of four trans people. This was a largely successful endeavour which elicited rich information, not least that some trans people feel extant language is inadequate to describe their lived experience. This is not to say that they could not speak in the research, but that what they spoke about was the inadequacy of words, perhaps specifically labels, when it comes to trans experience. As one might imagine, this left me in something of a quandary given that my aim was a phenomenological exploration of trans people's sexuality – which necessarily seeks to put into some form of words the worlding of trans people as relating to their sexuality. My hope is that my caveats above regarding my eschewing of 'grand narratives', my utilisation of direct quotes, and my careful contextualisation of the hermeneutic of suspicion will do some justice to my participant's voices and will not impose inappropriate meaning on the words they chose to use.

The other key area which was addressed after the pilot was that two of the participants were partners and, while prior knowledge of one another can be useful as we have seen above, it was felt this was too high a degree of intimacy for the group to function as a coherent whole as it instead seemed to leave a 'partnership' subgroup and a 'non-partnership' subgroup. For this reason, partners were explicitly excluded from the final group whose phenomena are analysed here.

Participants

Eleven participants elected to take part; several identified disabilities, but none felt that these would affect them in taking part or required any special provision to be provided for them during the research. Ethnicity and religion were asked as matters of standard demography, but did not arise in the data and are consequently not considered in depth in the analysis.

The participants (in order of presentation in the transcript and of course utilising their chosen pseudonyms) were:

Jenbury Handlebar-Smythe, who put their age in the 28–32 bracket and who identified as a Caucasian-Irish single female with autism, and as an Atheist.

Martin, who put their age in the 33–37 bracket and who identified as a white-British poly with wife + boyfriend + lovers trans man with hearing difficulties, and Pagan religion.

Charlie, who put their age in the 28–32 bracket and who identified as a white single female-bodied person with no disability, and Buddhist religion.

Mr Fox, who put their age in the 38–42 bracket and who identified as a white-British single/in poly relationship male-trans man with no disability, and no religion.

Cee Cee, who put their age in the 28–32 bracket and who identified as an African Scot single gender queer person with mental health issues, and spirituality (religion).

Scot Sam, who put their age in the 28–32 bracket and who identified as a white-UK poly[9] trans-man with no disability, and Pagan religion.

Sack Boy, who put their age in the 23–27 bracket and who identified as a white-British in an open relationship male with arthrogryposis, and no religion.

Haramit, who put their age in the 18–22 bracket and who identified as a white-Scottish Taken[10] trans (almost) male-bodied person with no disability, and no religion.

Tara, who put their age in the 33–37 bracket and who identified as a Scottish single female with borderline personality traits, and Roman Catholic (non-practicing) religion.

Jane Crocker, who put their age in the 28–32 bracket and who identified as a Jewish-Hispanic Polyamorous (2 current partners) female with clinical depression, and no religion.

Ezio, who put their age in the 23–27 bracket and who identified as a white-British single male with a (non-specific) learning difficulty, and no religion.

Notes

1 Note I am following Ricoeur (1970) and Langdridge (2007) in my use of the term here, rather than Giddens' (1984) use of the term double hermeneutic, to mean a social entity which is both being understood by social sciences and reciprocally understands social science (and so is changed by that understanding).

2 It may be argued that description is not properly a hermeneutic. However, I bow to accepted usage in this monograph and also note that it may be argued that, however rigorous my epoché for my attempts at pure description, inevitably a degree of interpretation will inflect (at least my choice of) descriptive terms.

3 Although the usual term suspicion may more usefully perhaps be described as contextualisation.

4 Van Manen (1997) is making a general point about experience rather than conceptualisation here. I have interpreted his "we" to mean humanity in its diversity, rather than a similarity of experience.

5 I'm including neutrois and asexuality here in the way atheism is, perhaps crassly, included under the broad rubric of 'religion'.

6 Of course I have the privilege to be out about my gender and sexuality – but if I do not make the point here then scholars less privileged than I may be forced to. And I firmly believe that when one has privilege one should use it for the benefit of those less fortunate.

7 Note the capital.

8 This is the practice of an adult identifying as a young child or baby for purposes of relaxation or sexuality. It is quite different from paedophilia in that it does not involve children, attraction to children, or coercion of any sort (cf. Richards & Barker, 2013; Richards, 2015).

9 Poly is generally short for polyamory – having multiple intimate partners (Easton & Liszt, 1997). Naturally, see Analysis and Transcript for the nuance of each participant's understandings of this term.

10 In a monogamous relationship.

Chapter 4

Analysis

The following analysis was undertaken using the design above and consequently each participant is discussed in turn initially. A picture of their model is shown for reference followed by a hermeneutic of description and then a hermeneutic of suspicion. Following this, themes from across the whole group are considered, again in the form of a hermeneutic of description and then a hermeneutic of suspicion. This explicit use of the double hermeneutic will, of necessity, include a small amount of repetition; however, the clear separation of description from suspicion should allow the reader to be more fully aware of the areas simply detailing themes which have arisen from the participants' explanations of their models, and those areas which I, as a researcher, have contextualised the material presented.

This structure of reporting is important because, as detailed above, trans people have historically been misused by the academy and I contend that the method of reporting itself can be marginalising if it obscures the individuality and humanity of the people who have participated. Thus, hopefully, this method of sequential reporting of participants in the analysis (rather than the usual method of a single narrative structure only referencing each participant when necessary; Moustakas, 1994) will allow the reader to see each person's unique experience rather than only as a chunk or chunks of information within a theoretical discussion, which risks losing the individual participant voice. Similarly, explicitly *showing* the themes separated from the imposition of theory will allow the participant's contributions to 'stand on their own' before I intervene. Hopefully the reporting structure used below will therefore ensure that any structural exclusion or dehumanisation is minimised.

Jenbury Handlebar-Smythe

Jenbury Handlebar-Smythe's themes included gender influencing sexuality, gender transition, and the use of colour to represent singularity and multiplicity.

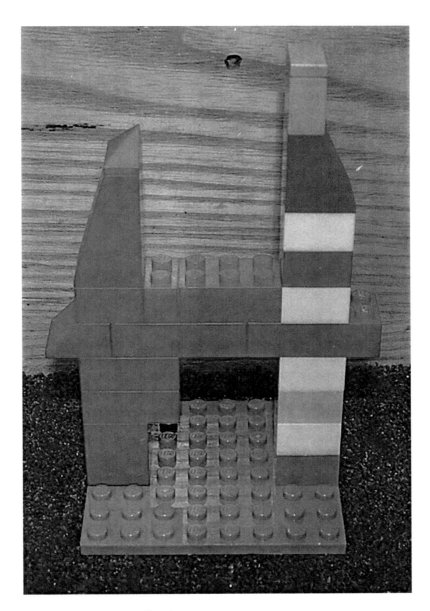

Figure 4.1 Jenbury Handlebar-Smythe

Hermeneutic of description

Jenbury Handlebar-Smythe made use of colour[1] to represent multiplicity stating that "the gender one is one solid colour" and "the one that represents sexuality is lots of different colours". Colour was also linked to limitation and expansion; "the uh sexuality one kind of fades to grey at the top . . . because, it's all gone a bit dry recently."

Jenbury Handlebar-Smythe also made reference to the influence of gender on sexuality stating that "my, uh . . . gender *does*, influence my sexuality" and "pretransition . . . during sort of sexual experience . . . my physical *sex* and how I felt sort of inside my head . . . there was kind of like *interference* . . . post, um physical, uh transition, it . . . provided more . . . avenues for enjoyment." This also reflected a necessary element of physical transition as an expression of gender as did her statement: "so, being aware of sort of my physical sex was previously distraction, negative, taking away from any experiences and these days is more of a, a positive, thing . . ."

This idea of difference pre- and post-transition – that is difference over time, marked by the event and process of transition, was referenced though noting how things were "pretransition" and "post, um physical, uh transition . . ."

Hermeneutic of suspicion

Jenbury Handlebar-Smythe appeared to be considering how her embodied self altered over the course of her transition in that her possibilities for sexual expression were opened up through her change of physical body. This is not to say that her sexuality per se changed (although there is evidence for this too in the literature; Auer, Fuss, Hohne, Stalla & Sievers, 2014; Cerwenka, et al., 2014; Coleman & Bockting, 1989; Lawrence, 2005; Rowniak & Chesla, 2013), but rather that, if we take her embodiment as being a physical-psychological entity, it allowed a fuller expression of her self and her worlding. Pearce (2014) characterises embodiment in this sense as:

> Embodiment implies that we are a totality of emotional, cognitive and physiological processes that are interacting dialectically and constantly to produce the constantly changing entity we manifest at each moment in time.
>
> (p. 108)

Embodiment in this sense might best be thought of as being expressed through an intertwined umwelt – eigenwelt (naturally with attendant überwelt and mitwelt). This will be culturally expressed, in that the expression of sexuality and gender varies across time and space – as seen above. This is reflected in Sartre's comment that "the nature of our body for us entirely escapes us to the extent that we can take upon it the Other's point of view" (Sartre, 1996 [1943], p. 358). Thus Jenbury Handlebar-Smythe alludes, both to her own wish to realise her sexuality through the medium of a congruent body, but also to a wish to be more accurately apprehended by the (culturally situated) Other whose point of view inscribes erroneous meaning upon it. Of course, Sartre is making the point that we cannot control, or even apprehend, the meaning the Other is inscribing upon us, but Jenbury Handlebar-Smythe appears to be refuting this in her sexuality-gender. She is, in a sense, saying that not all animals are equal in the degree to which the Other's apprehension escapes us and vice versa.

Of course, this is existential heresy. The idea that the Other can know us better subverts the notion of their being Other. Indeed, Smith-Pickard (2014) characteristics existential sexuality as that "we appropriate and are appropriated by the other" (Smith-Pickard, 2014, p. 90), thus keeping the Other intact through the need to appropriate rather than to meet (even Gadamer, 2004 [1960] suggests the fusion of *horizons*). However, I argue that it appears for Jenbury Handlebar-Smythe that the intersubjective binding of being-in-the-world-with-others (Heidegger, 2008 [1962]) means that we can enhance this intersubjectivity though our comprehensibility – in this case in an embodied manner. Perhaps the message for counselling psychologists here is that this linking of sexuality to gender to gender expression is part of self-expression and so comprehensibility within the social world. This means that understanding this complex linkage of the elements of sexuality and gender are a key part of our understanding (and so relating to) trans people and their embodied sexuality.

Of note is that Jenbury Handlebar-Smythe characterises her pretransition sexuality as "distraction" which we might read as inauthenticity in that she is distracted by a part (yet not a part for her) of herself. That one should be distracted by what is a key part of the self for many people (and indeed which Merleau-Ponty states is an integral part of the self; Merleau-Ponty, 2002 [1945]) suggests that the distractor (in this case disembodied sexuality) is being cast as an (albeit internal) Other. In this sense it is, as it were, a fragmentary I-Me form of relating (cf. Cooper, 2003) to this 'part' of the (not)self where the self is not regarded as coherent and so the incongruent aspect is split off. This may smack of Laingian psychic dis-integration, but recall from above that with trans people the body is not coherent with the brain/mind (and so then on to social intersubjectivity), rather than the person not being intersubjectively interrelated with society a priori. For many trans people however, and for Jenbury Handlebar-Smythe as we see in her transcript, bodily coherence brings about social coherence – as least as regards sexuality with "more avenues for enjoyment."

Martin

Martin's themes included being unique, overcoming barriers, time and the process of transition, and the gaze of the other.

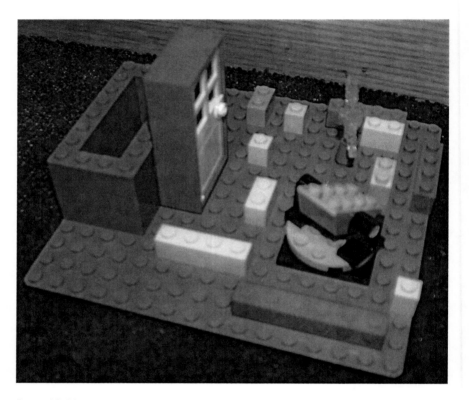

Figure 4.2 Martin

Hermeneutic of description

Martin made reference to being unique stating that "I've got a snowflake, because each one is unique . . . and that is definitely me", and that "I realised that I could be unique, as a boy." In a similar way to Jenbury Handlebar-Smythe, Martin used different colours to represent multiplicity: "lots of different colours because there's lots more in terms of my identity rather than just being this one boy." This was also reflected in his explanation of (and explicit knowledge of) the different parts of his identity and practice:

> "I identify as queer and I think that's a *(laughs)* really good way of explaining it, because it doesn't stay in one place or space, so my gender identity is

queerish, my sexuality is queer, my sexual orientation within that is queer, my um, the way that I *have* relationships is also, could be seen as queer, so that kind of fits within that."

Martin also noted a barrier (in the form of a wall) which an epiphany (represented in the form of a door) overcame, stating that "The blue thing yeah – is um, is me kind of bricked in, and it's specifically blue because I am supposed to be a boy, and I am supposed to do boy things, which is blue." But then noting, "Um so this is kind of pretransition and pre . . . discovery of me . . . the door represents that kind of line, so you come through the door and the wall bits are now exploded out . . ." This explosion, he explained, was where he had an epiphany: "I don't care what sort of man I'm seen as, as long as I'm seen as male, although, (*laughs*) I've evolved in terms of my identity since then, but as long as I'm seen as male then actually I can be whatever that means to me."

This overcoming of the barrier and his reference to there being a "process" since transition also references the place of time in Martin's understandings of himself.

His use of "what sort of man *I'm seen as* . . ." also references the gaze of other people in how he understands his identity as independent from them ("I don't care . . .") but also necessarily in reference to them.

Hermeneutic of suspicion

Martin poses clear questions to the orthodoxy of labelled identity taxonomies and so understandings. He, like Jenbury Handlebar-Smythe, makes reference to multiplicity rather than the dyadicism of male and female and the associated sexualities of heterosexuality and homosexuality. In this he implicitly references the postmodernism of Butler's (1988; 1999) deconstructions of gender and sexuality away from neatly explicable entities and into queer ontology, which troubles both traditional gender and sexuality categories, and also the very notion that such categories exist. Indeed Martin explicitly references being "queer" in various ways (as in the quote above) on several occasions. Notwithstanding this, he is also aware of how others (Others?) might see him and disavows their power to 'appropriate' him (Smith-Pickard, 2014) as a certain sort of man, provided he fits within the broad label of male in their minds, and further states that he has moved on from that position now too.

This is an important point for counselling psychologists. Words, labels, have great political power – from the intimate sphere (including within one's own mind) out to the widest of political spheres, having a label to put on an identity brings with it possibilities for the acquisition of power and control over one's own identity – and so place in the world. For those people who identify as cisgender and heterosexual, these labels may have been given at birth and so never have needed to be acquired by an individual for themselves. For trans and non-heterosexual people (who may be trans of course) labels must be acquired.

But in the acquisition, work must be done to see the points of fit and the spaces of disjoint from common stereotypes. Here Martin claims the label *Male* just as many trans men do, but also recognises that there are many aspects of his being-in-the-world which are specific to him. He continues: "As long as I'm seen as male I can be whatever that means to *me*"[2] thus reinforcing the primacy of his own conception of male for him – rather than a received delineation from others, be it media or wider society. This is at odds with commentators, mostly from the psychoanalytic tradition who suggest that trans people are mostly concerned with stereotyped fantasies (e.g. Chiland, 2005). In contrast to Chiland and others' erroneous conceptualisations, it is more often the case that trans people – having had the time for consideration detailed above – will come to nuanced views concerning gender much as Martin has done here. Trans people may, of course, go through a stereotyped (pseudo-authentic) stage when trying on identities at the start of the realisation of their gender (Richards & Barker, 2013) – but then, of course, cisgender people do this too, for example during adolescence.

Time is another theme which occurs within Martin's explanation. He *recalls* the epiphany he has while viewing the sunrise that he could be his sort of man, he speaks of his evolving identity – thus identifying transition as being a process across time. The idea that transition takes time is rather trivial of course. However, within that triviality is the more complex notion of the way people's pasts and futures are wrapped up together in an ever-evolving self-in-time. Martin references a memory of a plan for the future – his being is still emerging from the recollection which he carries with him for how he may be in the future. This sort of existential understanding of time (cf. Cox, 2009) can usefully inform the understanding of transition over time as being not as a series of static sequential events – but as an ongoing iterative and retroactively iterative process which continues after transition. Again, it is useful to be careful here, for this is a specific trans example of a process which people – trans or cisgender – undertake with regards to all manner of events, not merely transition. There are, after all, a great many transitions in all sorts of domains one might undertake. This is not 'something trans people do' which should be attended to when seeing trans clients only, but which has wider application for the practice of counselling psychology – perhaps we all have "[a] door [which] represents that kind of line"?

Charlie

Charlie's themes included change over time and the overcoming of past barriers, the hope for growth and personal comfort, and a consideration of choices.

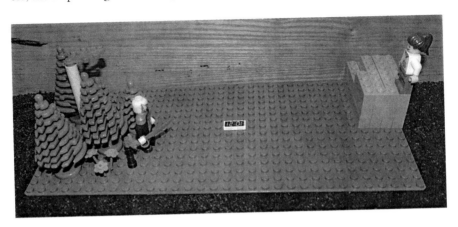

Figure 4.3 Charlie

Hermeneutic of description

Charlie also made mention of there being a "process" and the notion of time – going so far as to include a clock in the middle of their model.

Charlie also used colour to represent limitation, although in contrast to Jenbury Handlebar-Smythe, who used grey to represent a lack of sexual contact, Charlie used it to refer to "I suppose a sexuality that I have had, that I have, told was supposed to be a certain way and a sexuality and a body that I've never connected with so I avoided it pretty much all together."

Charlie also referenced limitations through the form of a "kind of a grey blank wall" but went on to express the hope that "if I have a body that I'm more comfortable with then the trees and the flowers on this side represent that I might be able to *grow* and kind of flourish a bit further down the line." This again referenced the notion of there being a process in time which included the hope for growth and also personal comfort.

This use of time was reflected in their statements that "I feel like I've lost a lot of time I suppose, I'm [*early thirties*] now. Um, time I've uh, I'm waiting for my appointment for the Gender Identity Clinic in [*place*] so it's the time now and the patience of having, having to wait. Um and at [*early thirties*] I know that the time that I have ahead of me and the rest of my life and how I want to live with that so."

There was also, in the quote above, reference to a Gender Identity Clinic as being part of the process necessary to the growth Charlie was hoping for, and the time involved in attending there.

Hermeneutic of suspicion

Charlie's primary themes concerned growth and, necessarily, time. I'll not needlessly reiterate the consideration of time above, but simply note that the wider philosophical understanding sketched above applies here too. The notion of growth, however, perhaps bears further consideration. Existential growth or potential had, until the second World War, seemed rather acontextual – for example Nietzsche's (1882) Daemon offered the opportunity to live one's life again and be praised or cursed for so doing. This is reflected, and perhaps updated, in the modern retelling of Nietzsche's Daemon in the popular television show *Red Dwarf* episode "The Inquisitor" (Naylor, May, Grant & Naylor, 1992) wherein a self-repairing replicant travels through time deleting people who have not lived a worthwhile life and replaces them with people who never had a chance to live. The difference between Nietzsche's Deamon and the Inquisitor arises in that the Inquisitor will only delete you if you fail to fulfil your potential, not if you fail to hit some universal marker of what constitutes a 'worthwhile life' (Richards, 2017c). A moment's thought reveals that this is far more profound – existentially it's not the hand you are dealt; it's how you play your cards.

For many trans people being trans means that there is a good deal of work to be done simply to get to square one, at least in regards to gender and sexuality, and this work, of course, precludes time for work on other matters. When Charlie speaks of "the patience of having to wait" he's waiting to (start to) play his hand, and in the final evaluation it's important to recognise that this is the case. For this reason counselling psychologists can perhaps usefully consider this potential starting position after their phenomenological inquiry into the context for the phenomena (as I have done here). This is because the temptation is so often to live with reference to the lives of others – as Charlie says; "glimpses of a sexuality I *could* have . . ." Indeed it may also simply take more time as there is more to do (gaining a coherent body for example). Therefore, while frustration with past change (or lack of it) is pertinent in such work, it can be useful to remember Schmich's (1997) wise quote: "The race is long, and in the end it's only with yourself."

Charlie also makes reference to the gender clinics in terms of the wait for personal growth. Much has been written about this context, mostly in terms of blogs and NHS overviews such as the *NHS Citizen Stocktake Gender Identity Services* (NHS Citizen, 2015), and some theoretical work concerning governmentality such as Davy (2010; 2015) and Sanger (2010). This will be discussed in the analysis below, but suffice to say here that they concern both [lack of] recourses meaning that there is a troublesome wait as in Charlie's account above; and also a query as to whether (and if so how) trans bodies and lives should be regulated by the medico-legal system. Of note here is that Charlie refers to "a sexuality and a body that I've never connected with", linking the two in that as he thought about gender he thought about sexuality too. Thus this governmentality of transgender from Gender Identity Clinics, while ostensibly about bodies, extends to sexuality for many patients as we have seen above and will see below, and dictates how many trans people, as for Charlie, may "*grow* and kind of flourish a bit further down the line."

Mr Fox

Mr Fox's themes included the positioning of his sexuality as strictly binary rather than queer. He made reference to other notions of sexuality impinging on his own, and explained that the process of his transition had allowed him to express his sexuality in what was now an ongoing exploration.

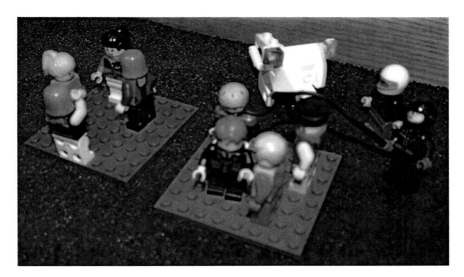

Figure 4.4 Mr Fox

Hermeneutic of description

Mr Fox made specific reference to his sexuality stating that it was a "butch motorcycle fetish type thing." He also exemplified some of the diversity of identity and opinion in the group, making clear that while he was "very confident and competent in understanding [queer theory]" he was not queer but rather bisexual (hence the two islands). He stated that "[queer] doesn't describe my experience *at all* in terms of sexuality. My sexuality is very binary, I have a very binary sexuality which is why I identify as bisexual and not queer."

His use of the islands also referenced multiplicity, but a multiplicity within groups (in this case "men" and "women") – rather than a purely fluid multiplicity. He voiced subtleties within this stating that he prefers; "Masculine men" and; "femme [rather than feminine] women." He also identified; "fetish and kink" as being part of his sexuality independent of the gender of the people he is attracted to.

He situated his understanding of his identity in reference to wider narratives regarding sexuality stating:

> "I feel there is a bit of a sort of a *tyranny of cool* in the sense that there is a pressure to kind of *be* pansexual, to be open to people on the *spectrum* of

genders and sexualities and that and kind of stuff, and that's absolutely cool if that works for you, but it doesn't work for me. I'm very much on those um binaries."

He also made reference to how his sexuality was inflected by his gender:

"I couldn't have sex with men, or relate sexually to men, when I was living as a woman. Just not possible to do. I *did* and it was rubbish, and I hated it and didn't do it for a long time. Now that I'm, you know, I'm a man and I'm kind of in my own masculinity that form of relating becomes possible, whereas it wasn't before."

Again noting that time and the process of transition (with the time of transition especially) was important: "pretransition this [*masculine*] world was closed to me . . .", but that this was also ongoing, "And now that I'm comfortable with my gender I can explore my sexuality fully in a way that I couldn't before."

Mr Fox made reference to the limitations of the medium of LEGO® stating that "They've all got bad hair by the way but I didn't have any control over that [*laughter*]." But later finding that the addition of a black leather hat resolved matters: "I can get rid of his rubbish hair now. Oh he's lovely!"

Hermeneutic of suspicion

Mr Fox again considered time and the nature of transition within the philosophical contexts detailed above – noting that he was unable to relate sexually to men before becoming one himself and thus intertwining sexuality and gender as others have done. It was clear that, for him, sexual expression with men must be mediated through his own masculinity and, especially, though his own *expression* of his masculinity – for example he states: "Now . . . I'm a man and I'm in my own masculinity that form of [masculine sexual] relating becomes possible." This sexual relating was wider than simply heterosexual or gay androphilic attraction as he spoke about "masculine energy" within the leather scene also. Of note though, is his telling phrase, the *tyranny of cool*, regarding queer identities where he, while noting he understands and accepts it for others, eschews it for himself. In this he rebuts Butler's (1999) philosophical deconstruction of gender (and as I argue here, sexuality therefore) in that his sexuality is dyadic rather than multiplicitous. Indeed, he specifically references queer theory as well as queer identities, stating that he understands it, but disagrees with it for him personally.

Of course, Butler's postmodernist (and indeed poststructuralist) arguments regarding gender and sexuality differ from Merleau-Ponty in that for Merleau-Ponty sexuality, separate from gender, permeates intersubjectivity, whereas for Butler sexuality, and especially gendered sexuality, is secondary to a form of performative gender within a (social) context. Because the meaning of gender changes according to time, place, and person, Butler argues it doesn't have an inherent a priori meaning, and certainly isn't linked to biological sex. This may be taken further to give a postmodernist read that gender and sexuality in this context have *no* discreet coherent nature outside of power relations in which they are (temporarily) constituted. Butler (1999) follows Foucault here stating that "[Foucault] understands the category of sex and of identity generally to be the effect and instrument of a regulatory regime" (p. 137) – in that regime gender, especially being female, is created though power relations wherein certain people are inscribed as women, or 'not men'. This is why Irigaray (1985 [1977]) states that women's sexuality is derived from men's. The difficulty here, of course, is that we have to use labels (words) such as 'women's' which might seem to have a reductionist meaning even though I do not intend that to be so. Nonetheless we therefore have two understandings of sexuality which are pertinent – the Merleau-Pontyian intersubjective and the Butlerian postmodernist.

However, Mr Fox's understanding of *his* sexuality appears to be at odds with both conceptions as his binary orientation also includes masculine (leather) sexuality which transgresses the strict bounds of heterosexuality or gay sexuality, in that it falls, at least partly, outside them as a separate entity. This complex inter-weaving only makes no sense if we look at it from a logical standpoint (that this entity cannot *not* be that and at the same time also be it). However we are explicitly considering the deconstruction of positivist viewpoints by including postmodernism, and so recourse to a meta-positivism in considering this epistemology seems disingenuous. Thus there are two options: (1) That Mr Fox is eschewing queer identities for him while including leather masculinity within his masculine sexuality, or (2) That he both has a dyadic masculine sexuality and a 'queer' (read postmodern) masculine leather sexuality as part of that – though he does not name it so. Philosophically these are equally valid, so perhaps we might use ethics as a final arbiter – given the argument above about appropriating trans people's voices: Mr Fox states he is *not* queer – it is therefore not for me to say he *is* from my comfortable seat in my academic ivory tower. Thus he has a bisexual sexuality within masculinity and has leather as a part of that. Simply that.

While identifying within a binary conception of sexuality Mr Fox also, like others, links sexuality to gender noting that he is attracted to "masculine men" and "femme rather than feminine [women]". While some people have a sexuality which is independent of a gender of attraction, or a personal gender (e.g. BDSM or infantilism; Richards & Barker, 2013; 2015), for Mr Fox and others the two are fundamentally intertwined. Further, Mr Fox made clear, again as others did, that realising his gender in the world was a key aspect of his sexuality becoming able to be established and acted upon. In the simple sense this would obviously affect who can do what sexually and with whom – what means one has to appropriate the Other if you will. But in the subtle sense offered in the existential sexuality of Merleau-Ponty in which sexuality is "a fundamental element of encounter and intersubjectivity" (Smith-Pickard, 2014) and where "as an ambiguous atmosphere, sexuality is co-extensive with life" (Merleau-Ponty, 1996, p. 169) something different occurs. Mr Fox's (emergent) sexuality is seen as a key part of his (inter)subjectivity and his gender is a key part of that – as he states, "in my own form of masculinity . . . relating becomes possible".

Cee Cee

Cee Cee's themes included multiplicity of gender and sexuality, with sexuality relating to two groupings of masculinity and femininity. They also expressed tiredness at living within societal expectations and made clear that this tiredness was not due to any sense of confusion on their part, but was instead to do with the trials of living within a society which is confused about them.

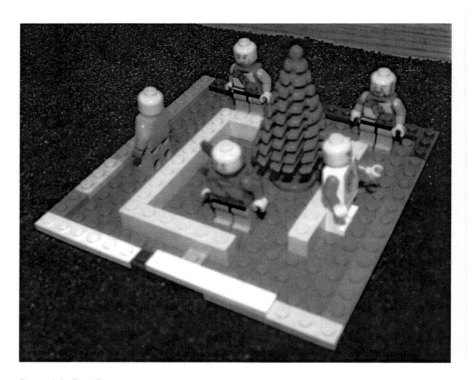

Figure 4.5 Cee Cee

Hermeneutic of description

Cee Cee identified as "genderqueer genderfluid" and recognised multiplicity within this: "whereas for me I feel . . . I neither feel female or male. I like playing around, but with *all* types of images of masculinity and femininity." This multiplicity recognised rough groupings within it, especially around "masculinity and femininity" which led Cee Cee to define as "Bisexual" – however the use of "*all* types of images of [masculinity and femininity]" suggested that bisexuality here was not being used in a strictly binary sense.

Indeed, Cee Cee recognised their identity as being in a discursive environment which was perhaps not fully reflective of them: "If I spent every single time saying no I'm not I'm a girl, no I'm not I'm this de de de. You know, I'd be worn out by now. So it's kind of I accept things from society, but sometimes it's out of convenience rather than because I'm actually ok with it." Cee Cee also made reference to the significance of bodies and representation of gender here: "if I've got really very short hair I'm treated as male, assumed to be male. If my hair is a bit longer I've got earrings in I'm assumed to be female."

Cee Cee also referenced nature as hope (for a change) in order that they "would love just to be . . . Cee Cee. Or and if I feel like being Cee Cee, my first name, but had the um choice to use a different name if I want to, um and be sexually free . . . of labels, sexuality labels."

This hope to be free of labels and wish to be free of societal expectations, or to be socially intelligible while being themselves, was represented by a barrier in the form of a fence and a wall – the living with which Cee Cee stated was tiring. Cee Cee was careful to point out that this difficulty was not due to confusion on their part – rather that it was difficult to deal with society's confusion: "I want to, um and be sexually free . . . of labels, sexuality labels. And be free of having to define my gender either way. But this *does* represent . . . a confusion. But not a confusion for what I feel like and what how I see myself, but external society's assumptions about me, can just be too, too heavy sometimes and it's just . . . yeah psychologically it can be very demanding. That's it."

Hermeneutic of suspicion

Cee Cee makes especial reference to labels and being labelled by others, finding the assumptions associated with this to be "psychologically very demanding." Of course, the psy professions can sometimes be seen as reflecting, or as part of, the society from which these demanding assumptions arise and it is notable that the phenomenological approach of counselling psychology attempts to avoid this through viewing things as they 'are'. Nonetheless Cee Cee's lived experience is just that, in general, people are unable to meet Cee Cee *as* Cee Cee because reliance on already established labels makes this difficult – indeed in my avoidance of using gendered pronouns here contemporary language somewhat struggles for the unfamiliar.[3] Butler (2005) considers this in *Giving an account of oneself*, where the very notion of being fully comprehensible in one's account of oneself to others is questioned due to the fact that we are necessarily constituted as 'selves' in childhood prior to our full awareness of what that means, and further "The language with which we communicate means that the 'mineness' of life is not necessarily its story form. The 'I' who begins to tell its story can do it only according to recognisable forms of life narration [labels]" (ibid, p. 52). Thus everyone is trapped in being somewhat inexplicable through not having a language which is at once both reflective of our unique experience and at the same time communicative to an Other of that experience. In the case of non-binary or genderqueer experience, as with Cee Cee, it may be argued that language allows still less of an account to be given. This leads to being even more marginalised – and we are aware that being in a minority can be psychologically stressful (Fiske & Taylor, 1991; Sherif, 1956) and that members of minority groups can be subject to what Sue (2010) calls *microaggressions*, wherein everyday interactions can become trying through social scripts not recognising people from a given minority. Once again, we butt up against the constraints of language as a poor tool for intersubjective relating, but unfortunately it is one of the very few tools we have, and the usual one for translation of non-verbal relating and identity in its recounting.

Perhaps in line with their subtleties of gender identity, Cee Cee also separates out their sexual attraction for males and masculinity as well as for females and femininity – rather than simply assuming an elision between male and masculinity or between female and femininity. Cee Cee is clearly aware, however, of the cultural signifiers of each, referring to having earrings as meaning they will be assumed to be a female, for example – but determining not to challenge people all of the time as this would be psychologically exhausting. Again, here we can see that philosophy is contextualised within lived experience. Cee Cee is perhaps meeting many philosophical criteria of existentialism in that they are not claiming gender as a fixed entity – as a *given* (Cohn, 2014 [1997]). In this case this is not at odds with their internal identity either, as it so often is with people who identify as 'a man' or 'a woman'. However, Cee Cee must live in the world and as such their reality is constrained. Consequently, they choose when to foreground their non-binary identity and when not to. This is a useful consideration for clinical practice, where philosophy and the lived experience of the client may be at odds and we don't want our clients to be "You know . . . worn out by now."

Scot Sam

Scot Sam's themes included adaptation within the medium of LEGO®, a recognition and overcoming of a barrier placed upon him by the world and culture, change over time, and a move to a more positive place.

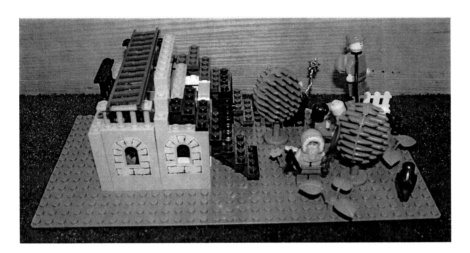

Figure 4.6 Scot Sam

Hermeneutic of description

Scot Sam found some limitations with the medium: "[the mini figure[4]] *inside* is um the closest thing to a girlie LEGO® thing that I could find" which he appeared able to overcome though using the figure as a jumping off point for the explanation. He also skilfully used the items as metaphors: "the sort of girlie figure in there is sort of sandwiched between two chests [*laughs*] and a skeleton [*laughter*]."

Scot Sam also used walls to reference a cultural barrier, "the fortress thing kind of represents the constraints that were placed on me by the world and the culture in which I live", and an embodied barrier, "the way I was *constrained* from being able to do that by having the body that I had."

Scot Sam also referenced time, stating that now "It's brilliant and really exciting and that's kind of where I feel I am now in comparison to where I *was*."

This change over time was linked to nature – a "garden" – being a positive environment where Scot Sam was able to express himself including the multiplicity of "a mixture of kind of different gendered figures in different ways", and a variety of sexualities: "some of them have like whips, some of them have, kind of dykey, some are fluffy girlie, some are S and M leather men, it's kind of a bit of a mixture." These were "not that deep."

Hermeneutic of suspicion

Scot Sam linked his body to cultural constraints – embodied constraints if you will. In addition, he identified a number of different identities which were available after transition: "a mixture of different gendered figures in different ways and . . . everyone's having a party and it's brilliant and really exciting and that's where I feel I am now." Unlike some of the other participants, Scot Sam didn't find this theme of multiplicity to be culturally inexplicable – simply that he couldn't access it in the body he previously inhabited. He used the word *constrained* twice and the word *contained* also, implying that he was aware of this multiplicity beforehand, but could not express it until he had made a physical transition. This is the common discourse of X trapped in Y body (Wilchins, 1997), although in Scot Sam's case it was X(trans man + various gender and sexuality forms) trapped in Y(female) body.

It is notable that Scot Sam explicitly notes various sexuality forms: kind of dykey, fluffy girlie, S&M,[5] leather men – some of which have necessarily gendered components and some which do not. Thus while Scot Sam required a personally congruent body in order to express his sexuality it was not as an objectively necessary part of these forms of sexual attraction, but rather because it was necessary *for him*. This is a slightly different take on the considerations detailed here with other participants which noted that some sexuality forms are only explicable for certain genders, and that sexuality may be taken as postmodernist (Butler), or as a part of intersubjectivity (Merleau-Ponty). While all of these, and perhaps especially sexuality-as-intersubjectivity, do fit here to some extent, Scot Sam simply wishes to express his sexuality, at least in part, in an embodied manner – once again his (gendered) body is an integral part of his sexuality. As Joseph (2009) notes:

> Existential phenomenologists describe intersubjectivity as if it is constituted through our embodied subject's interaction with another embodied subject of the same kind, overlooking the sexually specific differences of the two subjects – both sensory and morphological.
>
> (pp. 12–13)

Overlooking the heterosexism of this statement[6], Joseph's point is well made, in that embodied intersubjectivity is necessary if bodies are to be involved, and further that the specific attributes of those bodies matter. In terms of the sexualities Scot Sam delineates, they matter in terms of the physical capabilities, and also (perhaps tautologically given the Irigarayian formulation of gender given above) in terms of the gendered meanings and particularly meanings in terms of power relations which they inhere and communicate. These are for Scot Sam, as for many people, the "constraints that were placed on me by the world and the culture in which I live."

Sack Boy

Sack Boy's themes included attraction irrespective of genitalia, identifying openness in relation to his primary dyad, and change over time in relationship structure, but not intent or identity.

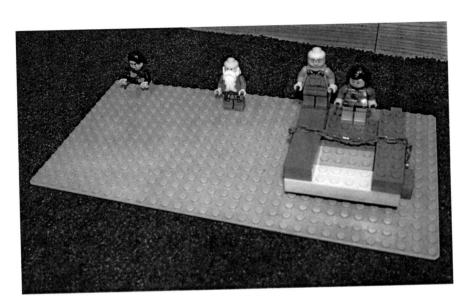

Figure 4.7 Sack Boy

Hermeneutic of description

Sack Boy referenced the two genders of him and his partner stating that they are "a man and a woman", but did not have gender as the defining feature of his sexuality, or indeed make reference to gender being related to sexuality in any way. He further stated of physicality that "I'm attracted to the person, and whatever's in their pants is . . . whatever." He included both a "man" (indicated by a beard) and a "sort of gender-queer, person with, no bits, uh who's genitals don't really mean anything to me" as possible partners outside of his primary dyad. He placed this dyad upon "a sort of pedestal" surmounting a "sort of open field sort of represents that openness [of an open relationship]."

Referencing change over time in terms of the form of his current relationship, but not his intent, he stated: "From being single for quite a few years I'm now in a sort of relatively stable relationship and I feel at home and a bit safe with her."

Hermeneutic of suspicion

Sack Boy viewed his sexuality through the possibilities afforded him by his relationship, both in terms of its current stability and also in terms of wider non-monogamies. This is reflected in Richards (2010), who showed that some trans people use non-monogamies as a means of foregrounding different genders within different partnerships. Sack Boy included two people in the field, one male and one genderqueer, and while Sack Boy's express intention with regards to his own gender was not explicit, it is possible that his mode of (gendered-sexual) relating would be affected by the gender of his partners. Indeed Smith-Pickard (2014) notes that "existential sexuality is a system of reciprocity whereby we fascinate and are fascinated by each other, we appropriate and are appropriated by each other, and what we desire is that the other person should desire us in return in mutual reciprocity." While, as stated above, I am unsure if this hard notion of 'appropriation' of the other is reasonable, there is some merit in noting how the fuzzy boundaries of our beings intersect (cf. Kosko, 1994), and how this intersection is likely to be inflected by the gender of the people involved.

Sack Boy also makes reference to how the safety of his primary dyad allows him to explore relationships more widely. As with all human relating, and perhaps especially sexual relating, the step into the unknown will necessarily be a leap to faith (Kierkegaard, 1980 [1844]) as the outcome can never be predetermined. However – within his model his primary partnership is literally 'raised up' to create a firm base from which such a leap into the (non-monogamous) unknown can be made. From within the tradition of counselling psychology the therapeutic space may be seen as such a base for our clients to make a similar leap to faith, and philosophically the place of such spaces within people's lives and within the therapy room – as well as such leaps themselves – is perhaps noteworthy, as we shall see below with reference to the gender clinics. Notwithstanding this, it might be nice if we as clinicians could offer somewhere to make such leaps where our clients too could, as necessary, "feel at home and a bit safe."

Haramit

Haramit's themes included careful, safe, change over time; fluidity; awareness of the gaze of others, but without the need to conform to it; a distinction between romanticism and physical sexuality; a freedom when being brought up; and a resistance to any chronological imperative for self-discovery.

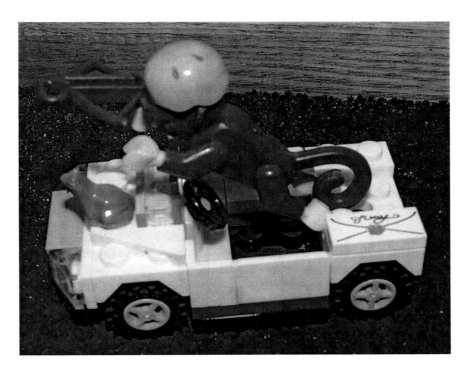

Figure 4.8 Haramit

Hermeneutic of description

Haramit referenced change over time and especially whether "everything is like . . . going to plan and stuff." This was in reference to "family and socialisation", and was presented as being done in a safe manner: "And it's wearing a helmet because, safety . . . obviously."

They also made reference to living in two worlds of gender and moving between them, with some difficulty, through the addition of a frog: "So it's kind of like they can, they live in sort of two different worlds. Kind of . . . Which is how I kind of feel sometimes with regards to . . . my gender."

They acknowledged the gaze of the other as not being personally important, but nonetheless inflecting their lived experience "because I don't really, I don't really care too much about my *own* gender or how people perceive me. But it seems that other people are a lot more interested in whether I am a boy or a girl or something else."

They also drew a distinction between physical sexuality and romanticism, stating: "I am *far* more inclined to form a romantic relationship with someone rather than physical."

They also identified as fluid, utilising a car as indicative of movement (rather than multiple discrete categories) in gender, sexuality, and beyond stating that "it kind of it kind of represents a bit of, fluidity and freedom, in kind of . . . everything . . ."

Haramit attributed some of this freedom of identity to "the way I was brought up was very, it was in a slightly more . . . there was less pressure on me to conform to one particular gender. Erm I was very free to, erm play with male or female toys or dress how I wanted to dress so long as I looked presentable."

This freedom from some societal constraints was still bound by time with Haramit stating: "I've never really felt too much in the ways of pressures starting trying to conform me into anything until I hit puberty." However, Haramit was able to resist this chronological imperative stating that, "I will discover who I am when I'm ready to discover who I am." And so "Erm, so I've always been quite free and accepting of myself."

Hermeneutic of suspicion

As with some others, Haramit also referenced time in his explanation, explaining that the pressure to conform to the expectations of the Others occurred at puberty – something which many trans people have recounted in their histories (Barrett, 2007) with greater gender latitude being afforded to people in their pre-adolescent childhood. Oftentimes puberty is when secondary sexual characteristics become visible (i.e. female-bodied children being required to put tops on and wear more gender-specific clothing). Again here we can see a link between gender and sexuality and the impact of society upon this. For many trans people this can be an especially distressing time as they are forced down an uncomfortable (wrong) track. Haramit, however, noted that they did not feel this pressure to conform from their immediate family, but rather from wider society. In this Haramit was similar to a number of participants who felt such an imposition. Haramit, however – perhaps because of their more comfortable upbringing – felt able to be 'amphibious' in terms of their ability to live in two different worlds without undue distress. Indeed their explanation was one of psychological robustness noting "I don't really care too much about my own gender or how others perceive me." In this way they were able to differentiate themself from some existential philosophy which suggests that they would necessarily be constituted by others. Instead they were I-I relating (Cooper, 2003), suggesting that they were constituted primarily by themselves in this way and were comfortable with that, stating, "I've always been quite free and accepting of myself."

This freedom, "a bit of fluidity and freedom in kind of . . . everything", is at odds with some narratives of trans development which suggest that, almost universally, there is a process of coming to acceptance of oneself (i.e. Bockting & Coleman, 2007) which is not posited for cisgender people. This heterogeneity of trans experience is important, not only here as we discuss themes in qualitative research, but, as noted above, also in quantitative research in which difference can be lost in the variance – as well as in the consulting room during therapy.

Haramit also notes that "I am far more inclined to form a romantic relationship with someone than physical." The common name for this, given their fluidity noted above, would be *panromantic*, although Haramit does not use this label – again possibly due to their preference for fluidity with labels being notoriously limiting on this as we have seen. This brings another aspect to sexuality – romance – which has not explicitly been mentioned before, but which nonetheless falls within, or adjunctive to, its domain (Carrigan, 2015; Richards & Barker, 2013). There has been little written about solo-romance in the way in which solo-sex (masturbation) has been written, but we might easily see how such a reconstrual could be made as a means of relating to oneself. Consequently, whether partnered or solo, we could see how romance might be a form of intersubjective relating which intersects with sexuality in the wider existential sense of the word discussed above, and in this way be respectful in our practice of people who are "inclined to form a romantic relationship with someone rather than physical."

Tara

Tara's themes involved her responses to her perception of a critical society and her concern that she must have an identity to navigate society.

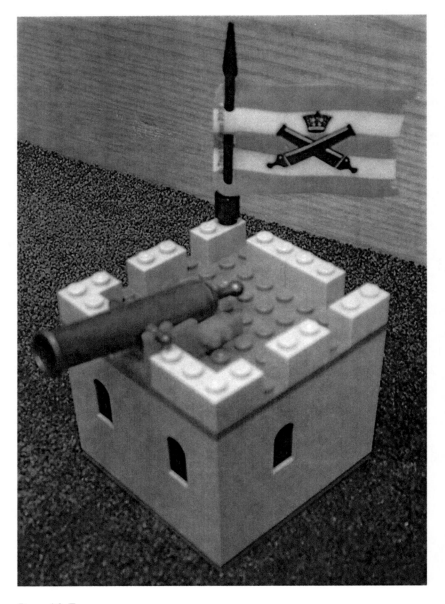

Figure 4.9 Tara

Hermeneutic of description

Tara recognised the part her online identity played in her life stating that she picked her pseudonym as "Tara because of my imagination, my original name that I think I ever used on the internet years and years ago."

She also recognised she had a barrier around her relating to her sexuality and gender which she represented in the form of a fort: "that's what it is, it's something I keep locked away from people and don't share with, um people." She stated the flag represented "[what] people see that they'll assume is what I am and who I am, but it's not what I am." And that in a similar theme the cannon, "is representing the fact that I can be quite, um, can be quite aggressively protective of my own sexuality and gender."

In this, the gaze of Others was apparent – "they'll assume is what I am and who I am" – as well as the need to navigate that gaze – "it's just what I put on to actually navigate society because you have to have an identity. Um, so it's I guess it's the one that's sort of forced on you by the assumptions in society on what you want to do, and the one that's most useful for navigating it." Tara maintained her control over her representation to society stating, "I let them see what I want them to see and that's about it."

Hermeneutic of suspicion

Tara spoke primarily about the 'fort' which she used to protect her from Others seeing her sexual identity. In speaking about this protection it is notable that she also avoided speaking about her sexuality directly as part of this research. She also spoke about the flag being what she wanted people to see – and again the flag was used to draw attention from her sexuality in the research. Nonetheless this was the phenomena presented in response to the research question and though this media. As Medina (2008) says,

> In the end it is the individuals experience that is key and the phenomenological approach must deal solely with the phenomenon that our [participants[7]] actually present.

Tara must, after all, wish to speak about her fort and flag as she chose to participate and not to redact the transcript. She states that she can be "quite aggressively protective of my own sexuality and gender" – that 'own' being important in that it is not subject to the gaze of the societal Other and therefore their approval or disapproval. One might argue that this is bad faith (Sartre, 1996 [1943]) in that she is not presenting her authentic self, however, of course, no one presents their authentic self all the time – it is simply a matter of degree. Notwithstanding this, Tara's sexual and gender self may feel too unsafe to expose to the view of critical others and so may feel safer hidden. In this she may follow some of the stages of coming out detailed in Bockting & Coleman (2007) or Richards (2011b) in which trans people feel the need to be discreet about their gender (and intertwined sexuality) until such time as their circumstances (both inter- and extra-psychic) allow for further disclosure.

She also notes that the flag is "not who or what I am, just what I put out to navigate society", once again citing the gaze of the societal Other as the restrictive constituent of her outward appearing. Note that she is still being constituted by Society in this way, in a very different manner from Haramit above who acknowledges the societal gaze, but opts to eschew it. As something of an existentialist I'm naturally drawn towards the notion of the waiter's apron, or the fin de siècle man's moustache which Sartre took such exception to, however, again I'm not sure this rings true. While Tara notes that her flag represents things which are "forced on you by the assumptions in society on what you want to do" she also notes that it is "the one that's most useful for navigating it." It might not be authentic, but it has utilitarian value. For me, it is useful to be wary of a sort of sub-cultural post-colonialism in which those of us working with marginalised communities impose possibilities derived from philosophy which may not be pragmatically viable. People do what they do according to their capacities, both personally and socially. Of course it makes sense to evaluate these from time to time, but I'll not sit here in my pseudo-Café de Flore and judge.

Tara also mentions the internet as being the place she first used her pseudonym. Since the advent of the internet it has not been uncommon that trans people have first come out online and inhabit cyberspace in their preferred avatar (Bornstein, 1994; Wilchins, 1997). This is troubling for some existential thinkers who suggest that we are necessarily physically embodied without recognising that in such instances our embodiment in the chair is simply a medium for accessing the internet and so, whatever adaptive technology one uses to access it, our presence is the same. Thus while authors such as Serning (2012) have argued that what is ready-to-hand online is constrained by our physicality, I argue that – for the gaze of the Other – what is ready-to-hand is simply the content of the online environment which also co-constitutes the person within it. Thus our self in such an environment might actually *be* a dragon, or a soldier, . . . or a woman. Tara, of course, suggests that she chose her (ready-to-hand) name "because of my imagination, my original name that I used on the internet."

Jane Crocker

Jane Crocker's themes involved a complex interplay between binary under-standings of masculinity and femininity and fluid notions of gender and sexual-ity. There was also a complex notion of adaptation over time while retaining latent parts of previous identities. Lastly there was reference to kink and how it crossed genders – but perhaps was manifest differently in each.

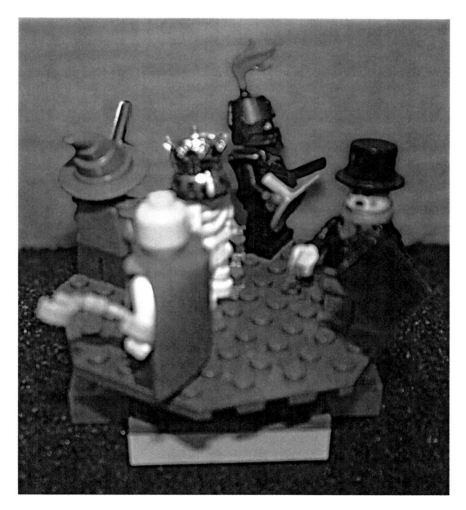

Figure 4.10 Jane Crocker

Hermeneutic of description

Jane Crocker used LEGO® mini figures to represent a complex interplay between a binary of masculinity and femininity, and a fluidity of genders and sexualities. She stated of her own transition: "I transitioned from, uh to put it in a very, what I would consider to be a binary way, I have transitioned from male to female", but also stated, "there's certainly a binary there in terms of femininity and masculinity but um, the rotation is what makes, uh the whole thing like *fluid*" and went on to say that this fluidity "can be like slow and pleasant or really, really fast and violent."

Jane Crocker also makes reference to the accoutrements of gender: "lipstick and . . . makeup." But intertwined with this is complexity as these figures also have a sword and magic. Indeed, Jane Crocker states: "The two more kind of feminine figures, um they both have like, um kind of beauty and they have magic and power and they and they're strong." Differentiating the masculine figures by stating that they have "armour which is more – I find – *defensive*" and noting of one of the masculine figures in armour that it "represents the times that I have used kind of masculinity as a kind of like as a *protection* both in the past and in the present, and so before and after, uh, transition."

The "past and in the present" here represents an acknowledgement of time passing, although not necessarily with change at the threshold of transition (in this matter at least) as masculinity was used defensively "before and after, uh, transition." Some part of a process over time was reflected in her statement: "both like what is past in my life but also like the remaining insecurities uh that have come with transition." This is evident in her reference to masculine power both being past and still latent, "kind of the dead king [the skeleton in the crown] is like some of the privilege I feel that I have lost that um um, that is gone and kind of like that past that is gone. But at the same time it is still there and has a crown so it is like, it has *power* so it's kind of like, you could see it as a sort of skeleton in the closet sort of thing."

Jane Crocker also made reference to kink, which crossed gender boundaries: "Um the other one, the noble man represents a kind of like a masculinity that is that I find more related to sex and hence the handcuffs, so kind of like kinky and such. Um um and so there's the [female] magician who also has the little bag of tricks that also represents like um kink and stuff and toys and such things."

Hermeneutic of suspicion

Jane Crocker made reference to both the gender binary and fluidity in her model. Of the binary she mentioned the accoutrements of femininity perhaps nodding to de Beauvoir's' famous quote, "One is not born, but rather becomes a woman" (1997 [1949], p. 301). However, she also referenced the sword as an accoutrement of masculinity, suggesting that – in a departure from Irigarayan philosophy, but arguably in line with Butlerian – both male and female are somewhat culturally constructed, rather than only femininity being in reference to masculinity. These are, of course, cultural signifiers which will differ cross-culturally in terms of their place in personal intelligibility within a culture.

Notwithstanding this, Jane Crocker undertakes a complex move in situating the gender binary on a turntable to represent fluidity. Again something which cannot be reduced either to logical positivist or postmodernist philosophies is represented. It is both binary *and* fluid – and I cannot allow myself to simply suggest that this (on a meta level) is a postmodernist deconstruction of binaries as this would privilege that philosophical position in a way which Jane Crocker clearly has not done. This appears to need a new philosophy (or more likely one I am not aware of) – the closest in my mind being Zen Buddhism, in which the apparent paradox of the binary and the non-binary are simply different facets of an underlying reality which is unknowable (Suzuki, 2011 [1970]). This foray into philosophy is important because phenomenologically it fits the present-ing reality – to impose either a logical positivist or postmodernist philosophy through misapplication of power would be inappropriate here and, by exten-sion, within the consulting room.

Jane Crocker also makes reference to the power inherent in masculinity with her 'skeleton king' representing the hidden power which she previously accessed and indeed since transition also accesses. Although acknowledging that the female figures are "strong" she also sees masculinity as being "more defen-sive", which she represents by giving her mini figures armour. This vulnerable-feminine defensive-masculine split is, of course, culturally understood back to (pre)history and is one of the complex areas which trans people must navigate in order to remain culturally coherent, while at the same time authentic. Serano (2007), for example considers the double bind of trans women who are required to be very feminine in order to defend their (questioned) femininity, while at the same time being told that being very feminine is not authentic as they are simply overly acquiring cultural accoutrements of femininity in order to buttress their (false) female identity. Conversely a trans woman taking on masculinity is also not authentic as they are not acting like a 'real woman'. Consequently the taking on of gendered characteristics not normally associated with their gender is arguably more difficult for trans people.

In utilising male figures in this way Jane Crocker appears to be separating identity from the expression, or perhaps better, utilisation of a gender form – and so is acknowledging the social encultured understandings of gender. Thus we have a separation of body, gender, and utilitarian gender expression as Jane Crocker states that she has "transitioned in a very binary way from male to female." This position then is effectively feminist in the political sense of the word. Again this is more complex than the traditional notion of trans gender as expression of an inherent internal gender (Benjamin, 1966). Jane Crocker does this, but is also able to express gender or gendered attributes – in this case masculinity – for their utilitarian instrumental ends.

Jane Crocker also references masculinity as related to (kinky) sex noting it is related to "handcuffs, so kind of like kinky and such." Kink or BDSM of course, are concerned with the consensual exchange of power (Taormino, 2012) and as such power relations are writ large. Easton & Hardy (2001; 2002; 2005) consider the gendered power relations in wider society we have been examining above, within the context of the explicitly negotiated BDSM environment, and the meanings inscribed upon gendered bodies in them – especially when a male top or dominant partner has a female submissive partner. This is because the implicit gender power relations within wider society may not have been negotiated within the BDSM relationship. Jane Crocker brings further philosophical complexity to this in that she is carrying over the masculine protective power assigned her at birth to the kink environment in an instrumental way, as detailed above. She also, however, has feminine figures associated with kink who have "a little bag of tricks that represents like kink and stuff and toys" such that she can represent her feminine self within kink environments. In this way she can represent both herself (female) and instrumental masculinity both within vanilla (non-kink) environments and also in kink environments – so upsetting the notion of the single inherent gender expression being all that is available to trans people.

Jane Crocker notes that power has changed over time in relation to her transition – hence the *dead* king. She characterises this as "some of the privilege I feel I have lost" from transitioning from male to female. And also acknowledges "what is past in my life [and] the insecurities which have come with transition." Here again, time – in the non-linear sense of the past and future inflecting the present and one another – is a key component of transition in terms of gender, identity, sexuality, and also [gendered] 'power'.

Ezio

Ezio's themes included a complex relation to time in which different aspects of a number of identities were foregrounded. They also referenced the past event of transition inflecting an engagement with the Bear[8] community which had occurred in the time since his transition.

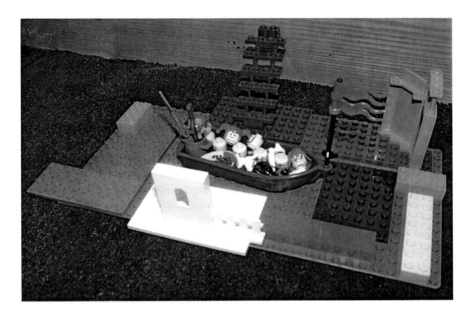

Figure 4.11 Ezio

Hermeneutic of description

Ezio utilised "lots of little different heads in with different faces" to represent different facets of his identity. He included a boat to represent some, perhaps fluid, movement between these:

> "it's a boat because it can travel between all the different bits um. And that's on a board with different colours . . . um, so really I've just sort of envisaged myself sort of going between these different parts and these are different aspects of my *life*. Uh where I sort of have different, or *act* differently or have different um ways of being myself in different situations."

He also recognised barriers, especially within the Bear community: "I feel that there *are* barriers there because I get to a certain point and I don't feel comfortable or say anything that's to do with um my trans history or um, like bits and bobs of *genitals* and different ways of how I feel about my *body*. Um so maybe yeah that's the um, the sort of barriers that I hit on. . . ."

Ezio also situated his gender in time, citing his trans reality as being in the past, albeit inflecting his lived experience in the present with his difficulties with the Bear community cited above. His use of "now" in "like the gay male sort of Bears which I am I very much consider myself a part of now" points to his recognition of time playing a factor in his identity – with a more complex relation to multiple, fluid identities needing to be foregrounded at different times: "But yeah the idea is at the boat will travel round to different ones at different times and be a certain way in a different situation. Uh but I don't feel that I can be all that at one point in time."

Hermeneutic of suspicion

Like other participants, Ezio references multiplicity in several ways: With regards to his identity – his "different parts"; how he expresses himself – how he "acts differently" in different situations; and also simply the different parts of his life. Again this might be regarded as rather disorganised in traditional psychotherapeutic modalities, but here it appears to represent the rather more reasonable position of presenting in a different way in different situations, much as we all do. For trans people (as one might imagine for other groups of people who are careful with their pasts such as indigenous people in occupied countries and members of persecuted religions) there is often a necessity to foreground certain identities in order to feel safe and to be culturally comprehensible.

Ezio particularly notes this in relation to the Bear community which, grounded as it is in gay male masculinity (c.f. Richards & Barker, 2015), Ezio feels would not be accepting of some aspects of his trans identity. He shows this in the form of a barrier, and includes various other barriers concerning other aspects of his desired life (which he can see through the window included in his model). He notes, "I don't feel comfortable or say anything that's to do with my trans history or um like bits and bobs of genitals and different ways of how I feel about my body." In this his embodied sense of self is acting as a barrier to the form of intersubjectivity he desires – he suggests that his subject will not be seen if you will, but rather an erroneous object will be perceived. Some existential philosophy would posit that we can never be truly seen by the Other – but again some animals are more equal than others in this regard, and it is a fairly universal desire to wish to be seen for who we are in our sense of ourself – rather than the facticity of the physical world, including the body habitus – we happen to have been thrown into. This is especially the case because (as Butler, 1999 argues) body parts come with culturally inscribed meanings which may not ring true to the person who has them – for example, the person in a wheelchair who is assumed to have a learning difficulty, the person with a penis assumed to be masculine, the person with long hair assumed to be feminine, the person with dark skin assumed to be dangerous, etc.

Ezio also considers time in his explanation, noting that "at some point the barriers will go" and again he is living in reference to non-linear time – here wrapping the future in his present. Tellingly he also notes that "The boat will travel round to different ones at different times and be a certain way in a different situation. Uh but I don't feel I can be all that at one point in time." That is, he has a multiplicity of elements which are distributed across time and circumstance. Of course this explanation is set in time and circumstance, and so we have an iteration of foregrounded elements with one explaining the others. This phenomena questions the notion of identity labels for gender and sexuality as anything but the most cursory of placeholders – politically vital ones as I have argued above and elsewhere (e.g. Richards & Barker, 2013; 2015), but perhaps not fully explanatory of Ezio's (or anyone's?) worlding which involves "lots of . . . different heads with different faces."

Group responses

Within the whole group, themes of barriers to appropriate interventions and especially a lack of support from Gender Identity Clinics figured largely. This was accompanied by a consideration of time and the process of transition, as well as a wish for support which was informed by the full range of trans experience – especially relating to sexuality – and which was accommodating of multiplicity and fluidity. There was also a key theme of embodiment relating to sexuality. As with the individual responses above, we will examine the responses descriptively – the hermeneutic of description – before turning to the theoretically contextualised hermeneutic of suspicion below.

Hermeneutic of description

The group discussed a range of topics with Tara commenting very early on that: "there seems to be a common theme of barriers . . . either ones people have put up themselves for protecting themselves or ones that people face for trying to access spaces. It's just the loss of freedom to move." The two parts to this – the barriers and the chronological adaptation of experience – were repeated throughout the group discussion. We will return to the key theme of barriers throughout, however with reference to time, this was evident when Scot Sam commented on "a past identity and a present identity, or a future identity." and Charlie spoke about "how I'm going to be for the rest of my life", indeed time, and specifically change over time, occurred repeatedly as key themes.

Concerning time and barriers, the relation to health professionals was a major theme in the group discussion – with frustration with the GICs being voiced by many participants. Mr Fox stated: "I realised what it was is that they'd stopped seeing us as human beings. They'd started to see us as *units* in a healthcare system to be processed, they'd lost sight of our humanity . . . we are so dehumanised I think as sexual beings in so much *else* of the way that society deals with us." Jenbury Handlebar-Smythe agreed, referring to clients in a gender service as a "product" and stating that "I certainly have the *strong* impression that no one who's involved in the medical care and treatment of trans people knows a damn thing about it. *At all.* Endocrinologists don't have a clue, the shrinks don't have a clue. It all, seems very disconnected from *our* realities . . ." This was a key theme which recurred throughout in terms of the limitations and barriers participants felt were imposed. For example, Jenbury Handlebar-Smythe said that "The GICs are far more 'No this is you must want *this* particular set of configuration and you must go all the way through to the end or you're not valid'. Um there's no sense of understanding that a big part of it for a lot of people is um becoming comfortable with who they are, what they are, um yeah and that isn't part of it it's about turning men into women and women into men." Cee Cee echoed this saying that they had to "follow the script" to get what they wanted in terms of physical interventions and stated that: "I think it's medical practitioners and psychiatric practitioners having a fixed idea of what a man is and what a woman is and – just do the swap." They also voiced concern with the limitations of GIC clinicians stating that they use "sort of the heteronormative model. And they're not, but the worst thing is that a lot of practitioners are not *aware*, of these biases that they're bringing into their assessments . . ." and consequently that "I never went to them for support or for guidance for that I went to my community . . ." Indeed Mr Fox stated: "In my experience the GICs that I have encountered are actually professionally negligent in the lack of support that they give you around sex and relationship stuff."

Notwithstanding this concern with the abilities and unexamined stance of GIC clinicians, there was a call for more support for trans people from professionals with Mr Fox stating that "The idea that any gender identity clinic in this country as far as I can perceive, from my involvement with them is offering *any* meaningful support whatsoever to people around sex and relationship stuff is laughable." Martin found the support "in terms of sex and relationships" offered by GICs to be "too medicalised" and was concerned that his therapist "Wanted to know from me, what the options were for men for lower surgery, rather than finding out through training channels."

Quite commonly in terms of transition, and again in relation to the GICs, the theme of *time* recurred – sometimes in the form of a 'process' – most often towards a more positive place. For example, Charlie referred to being "Early in this process [of transition]" and hoped to "grow and flourish a bit further down the line" noting that he was in his early thirties and was in the process of waiting for an appointment at a GIC. Martin used a door to represent pre- and post-transition with more colour afterwards to represent "lots more in terms of my identity" and spoke of having "evolved in terms of my identity"; Mr Fox stated that "pretransition this [masculine] world was closed to me . . ." and Jenbury Handlebar-Smythe: "Pretransition . . . there was kind of like *interference* . . . post, um physical, uh transition, it . . . provided more . . . avenues for enjoyment." Jane Crocker stated: "I have used kind of masculinity as a kind of like as a *protection* both in the past and in the present, and so before and after, uh, transition."

Alongside this, some participants spoke on the theme of feeling constrained by their assigned gender with Charlie avoiding his gender and sexuality as a "grey blank wall" until able to address it. Similarly Martin felt "bricked in" until transition when "the wall bits exploded out . . . [into] lots of different colours because there's lots more in terms of my identity." These constraints come from a number of different places, most commonly from societal expectations around gender (and sometimes from GICs perceived to be representing those expectations, as detailed above). For example, Cee Cee said, "for me how society sees my gender and sexuality and how I feel it to be, it's or most of the time is always in conflict. So I see myself as genderqueer genderfluid but society . . . if I've got really very short hair I'm treated as male, assumed to be male. If my hair is a bit longer I've got earrings in I'm assumed to be female . . . whereas for me I feel . . . I neither feel female or male." And (relating to GICs) "the heteronormative model. And they're not, but the worst thing is that a lot of practitioners are not *aware*, of these biases that they're bringing into their assessments." Tara similarly: "It's not it's not who or what I am it's just what I put on to actually navigate society because you have to have an identity. Um, so it's I guess it's the one that's sort of forced on you by the assumptions in society on what you want to do, and the one that's most useful for navigating it." And Mr Fox: "we are so dehumanised I think as sexual beings in so much else of the way that society deals with us." Haramit felt constrained only after puberty came: "I've never really felt too much in the ways of pressures starting trying to conform me into anything until I hit puberty."

Indeed many participants located the difficulties within society as specifically due a lack of knowledge beyond heteronormativity and consequently a difficulty with being comprehensible. Haramit stated: "I don't really, I don't really care too much about my own gender or how people perceive me. But it seems that other people are a lot more interested in whether I am a boy or a girl or something else." Martin stated: "as long as I'm seen as male then actually I can be whatever that means to me" and used the term *queer* to refer to himself. Similarly, as mentioned above, Cee Cee stated: "I see myself as genderqueer genderfluid but society . . ." With regard to the GICs, Jenbury Handlebar-Smythe stated of clinicians that "There's no sense of understanding that a big part of it for a lot of people is um becoming comfortable with who they are, what they are, um yeah and that isn't part of it it's about turning men into women and women into men." There was some resistance to this, however with Martin referencing the gaze of other people stating that: "Once I start on T[9] . . . I don't care what sort of man I'm seen as, as long as I'm seen as male", which perhaps links to the theme of change over time above.

Possibly in order to be intelligible, many participants did reference normative models of identity and sexuality, whether accepting or resisting them. For example, Mr Fox identified his sexuality as being "very binary" clarifying, "I identify as bisexual not queer" and stating that he was attracted to "masculine men" and "femme women". He expressed concern that "I feel there is a bit of a sort of *tyranny of cool* in the sense that there is a pressure to kind of *be* pansexual, to be open to people on the *spectrum* of genders and sexualities and that and kind of stuff, and that's absolutely cool if that works for you, but it doesn't work for me." Jane Crocker also referenced binary gender stating that "there's certainly a binary there in terms of femininity and masculinity" but going on to expand, "but um, the rotation [of the model] is what makes, uh the whole thing like *fluid*." And "I transitioned from, uh to put it in a very, what I would consider to be a binary way, I have transitioned from male to female." and Charlie spoke about being "in a female body." Perhaps because of the semiotic nature of the medium, participants used stereotypes to represent gender such as lipstick (Jane Crocker), beards (Sack Boy, Mr Fox), and some made reference to binary expectations elsewhere such as skirts for women (Jane Crocker) with Charlie commenting, "How in a female body you're expected, you know there is an expectation of the role you are supposed to play."

These understandings about culturally comprehensible signifiers of gender were also noted by Owen (2012) in their phenomenological research on trans. Owen states: "Because the realm of any meanings and cultural practices are intersubjective . . . [t]rans-sexuals (sic) appropriate pre-existing gender codes in order to express themselves like anybody else" (p. 210). However in the current research this was made more complex with a wide range of gender identities being held by the participants beyond only male and female. These included female, trans man, gender queer, genderqueer, genderfluid, queerish, trans-man, male, trans (almost) male. And a range of sexualities labelled including romantic, queer, kink, S&M, gay male Bear culture, bisexual, leather, dykey. There were also a range of relationship structures recognised including being single, poly, having a partner. A further mode of complexity was the mixing of commonly gendered items such as Jane Crocker's use of lipstick and a sword for one of her feminine figures and the notion of fluidity represented by movement which occurred in several models such as Harmit's letter, Jane Crocker's turntable, and Cee Cee's multiple people, for example.

While terms such as *Bear* implicitly linked sexuality and gender, some participants explicitly linked them. For example Jenbury Handlebar-Smythe stated: "My gender does influence my sexuality." Martin used the term *queer* to identify his "sexuality" and "sexual orientation" as well as his "gender identity" which he referred to as "queerish". Naturally, implicit links will be discussed within the Hermeneutic of Suspicion subsection below, but here it is worth noting also that there was a common theme linking embodiment to sexuality. For example, Mr Fox commented, "If you are trying to have a sex life with a penis that looks like Chewbacca[10] [*laughter*] that is going to affect your ability to have a functioning sex life. . . . You know trying to have, or given a blowjob, and trying to have that kind of sexual conversation with someone when you're trying to have to explain why your penis is covered in hair." And that "[GICs need to provide] *support* in terms of sex and relationships . . . if somebody doesn't even know what surgeries are available how can you then advise somebody on what it is that they then might want to do with what, what is available to do with those body parts, what you might want to get into."

This was not always simply that participants were not able to be sexual with their pre- or non-surgical bodies. While Charlie said, "I think for me a lot of it is, you know, *body* related", the necessity for a certain type of embodiment was both embraced and resisted with Martin stating that:

"I did enjoy my body but I repressed that because I wasn't supposed to. As a trans person I was supposed to hate my body. And that was what I got from the clinics was that I should not enjoy my body. I should be having lower surgery because there is something wrong with my body. Um there's not something wrong with my body. My head doesn't fit and I'm not comfortable with it at that particular point. But actually now I've had certain surgeries and I've had hormones I am no longer gender dysphoric but I am still trans."

Tara also stated that "if you indicate any enjoyment [with your body] you're seen as a pervert." Martin also expressed concern about the undue attention health professionals gave to physicality: "The first question I was *ever* asked every single time was 'So have you thought about lower surgery yet?'" Similarly, Sack Boy was frustrated that his contentment with his penis was not recognised: "It's like 'no you're not listening to me you're basically thinking like I've made a mistake because I want a small willy' [*laughs*]. And it's like I just don't think they could get it in their head that I would be happy with something that maybe biologically is under, under the average, but I'm more than happy with it." And "I um pretty much I would say I I've gone for metoidioplasty[11] because it suits me as a person my sexuality. Um I'm a bottom more much more than top so then I'm not really interested in penetrating someone." Thus sexuality and (embodied) gender formed a key intertwining theme in many participants' statements.

Hermeneutic of suspicion

As can clearly be seen above, the participants' responses were heterogeneous. Some participants identified within the gender binary and within heterosexuality, and others did not. Some participants were explicitly queer or non-binary, and some were perhaps implicitly so, with identities at odds with their body habitus. Consequently situating all of the participants within a single unifying notion or philosophy would be so procrustean as to do a violence to their contributions – and therefore naturally that will not be attempted here.

Nonetheless, there were some overarching contexts and themes which the participants referenced – whether through accepting or resisting them. One of the key themes concerned the inadequacy of the GICs – especially (and sadly ironically) with regards to sexuality and gender. It is notable that the participants chose to spend a good deal of their time considering this inadequacy rather than endeavouring to add to the knowledge they felt was lacking through the medium of this study. This issue will be considered further within the Discussion section below. A key model which may contextualise this here, however, is that for many trans people sexuality is dependent upon having a body which is an appropriate means of expressing that sexuality – and the link from their identity to that body is via the GICs. It follows therefore, that any discussion of trans sexuality is likely to include this vital – and apparently flawed – link. Consequently we might visualise this chain as shown in Figure 4.12.

For some participants this chain was in evidence as they understandably felt that they needed to have a body which was culturally comprehensible within

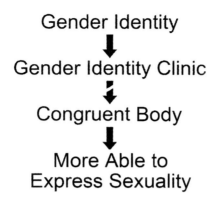

Figure 4.12 The place of GICs in trans sexuality

their explicitly stated sexuality – thus if one wishes to engage with heterosexuality one needs a partner with a body configuration different to one's own. Or if one wishes to engage with gay male Bear culture one needs to have a gay male Bear body. This is the commonly represented theme in the literature (e.g. Barrett, 2007) and it follows that people who are precluded from having a congruent body will be unhappy with it. Indeed this does seem to be the case for many trans people (ibid), but it is not the whole case. Martin noted that things were "in the support group that I set up . . . very much different because I *was* enjoying my body where the other people in it seemed like they weren't." Several participants felt that this discourse of necessarily hating one's body being a precondition of being trans came from GICs – Martin again: "I *did* enjoy my body but I repressed that because I wasn't supposed to. As a trans person I was supposed to hate my body." And Sack Boy: "The first question I was *ever* asked every single time was 'So have you thought about lower surgery yet?' I'd been very, very clear from the very beginning as soon as I knew it was available that I never wanted lower surgery". Thus for these participants physical interventions (via GICs) were more about enhancement rather than removing a deficit, or about addressing specific elements of their bodies – rather than addressing bodily dysphoria *in toto*. Both Tara and Martin noted, however, that this discourse of necessarily hating one's body was situated within trans communities as well as within the GICs:

TARA: It's just to say that when you are talking about the, um about not being able to enjoy your body when it comes from outside, well it comes from the community as well . . .

MARTIN: Oh yeah it comes from the community as well.

However this is not to deny the reality of some trans people's actual discomfort with the body. For example, Charlie said:

> "I think for me a lot of it is, you know, *body* related. And how, how in a female body you're expected, you know there is an expectation of the role you are supposed to play, and that has never been comfortable for me. But, so it's good to hear stories of people who have found other, other ways of being and ways to express that, and are happy with that, so that's good."

The difficulty which arises for many trans people then, is that in expressing either discomfort or comfort with one's body, the discourse of this is situated within a power relation – with the source of the production of this discourse being both the GICs and the trans communities. Foucault (1991 [1977]; 1998 [1976]) characterises this as a power/knowledge integration where knowledge (in this case whether one is comfortable) and power (whether such comfort is socially acceptable) is constitutive of discourses of this type, and arguably also constitutive of the actors (the participants here) also – as we have seen above with the participants in this study who have necessarily taken a stance in relation to it. This stance, one might argue, is aimed at being existentially authentic, in that the participants are arguing for the right to self determination – a *will to power* if you will (Nietzsche, 1968 [1895]) in which they are able to express their freedom and, crucially, to take responsibility for that freedom (Sartre, 2003 [1943]) without the GICs taking it from them through determining appropriate treatments. Indeed the reiteration of the difficulties with the GICs here, and the knowledge/power production so produced, might be considered to be a part of that freedom and responsibility.

Some participants appeared to suggest that this discourse of power/knowledge integration concerned a normative model of gender and sexuality, and often a specifically heteronormative one – as Sack Boy commented: "It's just um I think there is a lot of hetero heteronormativity . . . and they [the GICs] just presume that. 'Oh you want to be with a woman', and that is why . . . I just pretended [to the GIC] I did". And again participants reported embracing or resisting this – Jenbury Handlebar-Smythe:

> "but [GICs] were concerned about um trans women getting on hormones and then not having genital surgery. Oh yeah, they were creating a they were creating *she*men (*gasp in background*) was the term the clinician had used."

It was also suggested that trans people were telling GICs that they were heteronormative in order to access treatments (cf. Bockting, 2008), but in fact (as seen in this research) that they were not – Jenbury Handlebar-Smythe again:

> "[I'm] aware that [trans] people's relationship with gender tends to be . . . a lot more complicated, and, very much, the people who are happiest are the

people who know who they are and can get to the place where they need to be to be comfortable in themselves."

He also stated that:

"It was quite well known within the uh trans communities at the time, and I assume it's still the same, is that the um, the psychologists uh, are purely gatekeepers and here's what they want to hear. And that's what you tell them, because if you tell them anything else they won't let you through the gate, so they have this constant positive reinforcement of 'oh these people are all saying this thing and they're all checking off our list therefore anyone who deviates is obviously not conforming therefore not *really* trans.'"

Thus explaining how GIC clinicians were reinforcing heteronormativity and having it reinforced to them by their trans patients in a problematic feedback loop. Further, Cee Cee commented:

"I think that um what the experts [air quotes here] um, what influences how they see male and female will always be influenced by their own idea of sexuality, you know man's sexuality and women's sexuality. So sort of the heteronormative model. And they're not, but the worst thing is that a lot of practitioners are not *aware*, of these biases that they're bringing into their assessments and work that you're doing just now, us talking is really important that they get that."

Consequently one of the key elements from a counselling psychological perspective appears to be either a lack of reflexivity on the part of the professionals the participants have seen, or that those professionals were applying heteronormative practice deliberately – possibly as a result of having it reinforced by the trans people they saw. Either way, this was reported as being at odds with several participants' identities. This led to the common practice of telling GIC clinicians a certain (heteronormative) story in order to access treatments as Jenbury Handlebar-Smythe noted above and as Jane Crocker stated:

"Before I set foot [in a GIC] I had spoken to a *lot* of people that had been there that had been through it that had been through that system for many years to know what was wanted of me and what was expected of me and I did, I never deviated from that because I knew what I wanted and what I needed. Um, and so I did not, um I never went to them for support or for guidance for that I went to my community outside of that."

Other elements participants took issue with regarding GICs included a simple lack of knowledge. Jenbury Handlebar-Smythe: "I certainly have the *strong* impression that no one who's involved in the medical care and treatment of trans people knows a damn thing about it. *At all*. Endocrinologists don't have a clue, the shrinks don't have a clue." And Mr Fox: "I was trying to explain it to these very very eminent people who work with us *every* day and they could not get it and I thought 'Why can't they see this very obvious thing?'"

This lack of knowledge, and associated appropriate treatments had a knock on effect on sexuality as Mr Fox above had been trying to explain why penile hair removal was important for trans men as it allows them to receive a blowjob, for example; or Sack Boy who was frustrated that surgeons could not understand his decision that "I would say I I've gone for metoidioplasty because it suits me as a person my sexuality." This is more evidence for the link for some participants between embodiment and sexuality – or rather an embodied sexuality and fits with Merleau-Ponty's notion of sexuality as

> relationship to other persons, and not just to another body, it is going to weave the circular system of projections and introjections, illuminating the unlimited series of reflecting reflections and reflected reflections which are the reason why I am the other person and he (sic) is myself.
>
> (1996 [1945], p. 230)

To weave this "circular system" the circle must be intact. Perhaps because some clinicians have failed to see this, some participants felt that clinicians were no longer seeing trans people as people – Mr Fox regarding penile hair removal again: "

> "The fact that these men, and they were almost all men, there were no women there, the fact that these men can't get it. Why not? Why can't they get it? And I realised what it was is that they'd stopped seeing us as human beings. They'd started to see us as *units* in a healthcare system to be processed, they'd lost sight of our humanity. So think what was really important for me was that this was about, this is little *people* this is me as a *person* these are little people this is real human beings."

This "seeing us as real human beings" is, of course, the sine qua non of counselling psychological practice – meeting people as they are, rather than as a 'unit to be processed' – I-Thou relating (Buber, 1958) where we see people as fully people, and here integrating identity, gender, physicality, and sexuality together in nuanced (circular, intersubjective) ways (cf. Pratchett, 1998; Richards, 2017c).

Perhaps seeking such engagement, some participants felt that a greater amount of therapeutic time, presumably while being seen as a person, was needed. For example, Tara stated:

> "In that case it's the difference between what you see in the States people go through so much psychological counselling. We've maybe, people might have seen a psychiatrist five times and then they're sent off for pretty, relatively major surgery without actually having dealt with things."

Again such exploratory, rather than didactic or directive, practice fits well within existential-phenomenological counselling psychological tradition (van Deurzen-Smith, 1997; van Deurzen & Adams, 2011).

Of course, clinical practice from other traditions also continues to evolve. It should be noted therefore, that participants drew upon a range of experiences from different time periods. For example Jenbury Handlebar-Smythe stated that: "I transitioned at the tail end of the nineties and early two-thousands." Tara stated: "it was the late nineties that I first got involved and it was even worse back then, than it is now." And Cee Cee noted: "Friends of mine that transitioned late nineties early two-thousands talked about the very same thing of having to answer certain questions in such and such a way." Martin commented: "I started transition early two thousands." Jane Crocker spoke about her transition: "this was in two thousand and eleven." Consequently some of these experiences of GICs (but not, of course, of identity formed by such memories) will predate recent guidelines such as the *Good practice guidelines for the assessment and treatment of gender dysphoria.* (Royal College of Psychiatrists, 2013); the *Standards of care for the heath of transsexual, transgender and gender nonconforming people* (7th ed) (WPATH, 2011); and the *Interim gender dysphoria protocol and service guideline 2013/14*[12] (NHS England, 2013). However, for our purposes here this should not draw undue attention as the field is evolving at such a rate that practice will always be (one hopes) developing so that it has evolved from people's past experiences. In addition, the discourse concerning treatment by gender clinics is the phenomena – it is the thing being presented by participants as an important part of their current worlding. No matter when their personal experience of it, it informs and inflects current experience of living in the world. Indeed the discourse also informs and inflects the current experience of people who are attending clinics now or recently (as we saw with Jane Crocker) due to trans people communicating about it via the internet or face-to-face. Thus, while some aspects of trans people's experiences of GICs will become outdated, the discourse will remain current and important to attend to.

One of the key barriers to self-actualisation participants noted, and indeed modelled in LEGO®, was therefore the GICs. Another was societal opprobrium – although in referencing the heteronormativity expected within GICs participants may have felt this was part of wider societal heteronormativity as when Cee Cee commented: "I think I think it's medical practitioners and psychiatric practitioners having a fixed idea of what a man is and what a woman is." This is against the positioning of both those existential thinkers such as Spinelli (2014) and Cohn (2014) who cannot accept an "inflexible cultural grid" of gender and sexuality (p. 66) as well as thinkers such as Langdridge (2014) who accept a more rigid notion of a person's declaimed sexuality and gender, but commented that:

> For me, it is my duty to offer more, to use the weight of my authority and privilege not only to listen and understand but also to act as co-critic of the

heterosexist and homonegative world we inhabit so that my clients receive as much from me as I can possibly give.

(p. 172)

This wider societal heteronormativity is evident in how participants saw society as viewing *whether* they have a sexuality. If one assumes that within a narrow reading of heteronormative discourse trans people are 'really' of their birth-assigned gender, then it would follow that trans men are 'really' women and therefore don't have a sexuality, whereas trans women are 'really' men and there-fore are perversely sexual in identifying as women (cf. Serano, 2007). This is, of course, nonsense (Richards & Barker, 2013; 2015), but it does drive some societal discourses. Mr Fox again:

"I think, I think when I think about how trans people are represented in terms of our sexuality we're very, very *de*humanised. So it's either, you know, there's either the sort of stereotypes of, you know – and this is vile language and I don't like it – but kind of you know *she*male porn and that kind of thing or trans men, so we don't have a sexuality at all."

Thus heteronormativity is difficult both for trans people who adhere to het-eronormative societal rules, but are found wanting through being trans (Serano, 2007), and also those who wish to live outside of such rules and therefore have their gender (of whatever sort) questioned (Bornstein, 2004). As Cee Cee commented:

"I want to, um and be sexually free . . . of labels, sexuality labels. And be free of having to define my gender either way. But this *does* represent . . . a con-fusion. But not a confusion for what I feel like and what how I see myself, but external society's assumptions about me, can just be too too heavy sometimes and it's just . . . yeah psychologically it can be very demanding. That's it."

It follows therefore that the barrier is, in fact *against participants having a body and/ or a self which is congruent with their internal (sexual) selves*; (which may of course be any sexuality [or none] one might think of; Richards & Barker, 2013) – rather than against any particular body configuration or sexuality. The need is to be comprehensible and congruent within whichever body-sexuality-self the per-son has and wishes to have as it interrelates with their preferred Other (again, be that a person, or sexual practice, or both) and with society more broadly. Thus when Sack boy says, "I've gone for metoidioplasty because it suits me as a person my sexuality. Um I'm a bottom more much more than top so then I'm not really interested in penetrating someone", and Mr Fox states, "that kind of masculinity, that kind of very heavy, um, you know the kind of *leather scene*, all that kind of stuff it's a really powerful form of sexuality. Um and that was kind of closed to me because I couldn't have sex with men, or relate sexually to men, when I was living as a woman", these utterances may be from within the same philosophical frame.

This wish to overcome barriers and therefore be congruent, naturally occurs over time, and was another of the major group themes. As stated above, time in this sense is not unidirectional, but is rather composed of the past and future inflecting the present. The notion of transition is of course bound up in time, but it is not simply a transition from male to female or vice versa formed through time – or even from one gender (of whatever sort) to another. Instead it is a consideration of the whole of a person and how time is inflecting that person, infusing their being if you will. For example Ezio said, "a boat will travel round to different ones at different times." Certainly gender and sexuality, in the intertwined way we have been considering them here (and with whatever labels attached), form a key part of this self-worlding-in-time, but we must be careful not to limit transition to a matter of only gender in the simple sense. As Martin said:

> "And I remember if I started on testosterone walking along seeing the sun rising somewhere or other, and *just* that image has stayed with me as a kind of epiphany moment of once I start on T . . . I don't care what sort of man I'm seen as . . ."

This transition is also not necessarily from one unitary place to another unitary place, but rather may embrace fluidity or multiplicity – thus it is not a single unified step from one 'self' to another. Some participants demonstrated this through their models having multiple mini figures – sometimes grouped to form a rough set and sometimes not. Others reflected fluidity and multiplicity in the nuance of the transition, referencing growth and change rather than a simple break from one thing to another. This was reflected in the language used also – with identities such as queer being claimed as well as identities with nuance – for example Haramit was "*far* more inclined to form a romantic relationship with someone rather than physical." Others detailed varying sorts of BDSM, and Scot Sam, for example noted: "[the mini figures are] just sort of random they all have, or some of them have like whips, some of them have, kind of dykey, some are fluffy girlie, some are S and M leather men, it's kind of a bit of a mixture."

Notes

1 Please excuse the omission of colour plates in this monograph. Colour plates would have made the book prohibitively expensive, which would have lessened the number of readers. I felt that this would have done a disservice to the participants who so generously contributed.
2 Italics my own.
3 I could, of course, use Zie, Hir, etc. as gender neutral pronouns, although some readers may be unfamiliar with these terms (cf. Richards & Barker, 2013).

4 This is the name given by LEGO® to their small humanoid figures.
5 This usually means consensual erotic power and/or sensation exchange: Bondage and Discipline, Dominance and Submission, and Sadomasochism (BDSM)/Kink often shortened to S&M (Richards & Barker, 2013).
6 And note here that I am doing the onerous work many participants describe in attempting to make explicable non-heteronormative accounts in a heterosexist society.
7 Medina uses *clients* here, but – just as kata becomes kumite – so in my view the phenomenological method philosophically flows from therapeutic client 'research' to (nominally) non-therapeutic participant research.
8 The Bear community is a gay male subculture which involves hirsute males and evolved from blue-collar workers especially.
9 Testosterone.
10 Chewbacca is an extremely hairy humanoid from the *Star Wars* film series.
11 The surgical creation of a penis which is smaller than average for the cisgender population from the person's clitoris which has enlarged after the person has taken testosterone.
12 This is still extant at the time or writing due to political difficulties.

Chapter 5

Discussion

The participants presented a range of different themes with heterogeneity being perhaps the overarching theme. This heterogeneity was evident in both the information the participants gave about themselves and also in their relation to the themes which emerged. This rather belies the assertion made by Person and Ovesey in 1974 that "To know one [trans person] was almost literally to know all" (p. 18). Such assertions in the historic literature about the homogeneity of trans people (and indeed other minority groups) have, as we have seen, been overturned by the current literatures of which, it is hoped, this monograph will form a part.

One might assume, however, that in scientific research a finding of heterogeneity is a failing in so far as the object of research is to find themes which must necessarily have a degree of coherence or homogeneity. However, the nature of the research, and the epistemology that underlies it, are to see (in so far as is possible) the phenomena for what it is – and so heterogeneity as a (coherent, if ironic) overarching theme it is. Indeed, as can be seen from the literature review, this is not an unusual finding in this field. This intersects clearly with existential understandings, as Milton (2014c) notes, "for psychotherapists reductionist thinking is a problem as it cannot offer us the wider awareness that human science needs and existential thinking can contribute to" (p. 11). Indeed Manafi (2014) suggests that the authors included in Milton's (2014b) edited collection *Sexuality: Existential perspectives* "Give voice to the complexity, uncertainty, ambiguity, diversity and plurality of the most intimate, and at the same time public, aspect of our being – namely our being-in-the-world sexually" (p. xi). Heterogeneity then, is both acceptable within the existential tradition, and also appears to be a tenable finding from this (and other) research.

Notwithstanding this, there are some tentative themes which have nonetheless been found in the present research. These primarily concern *Barriers, Time, Reference to multiplicity or binary identities*, and *Gender Identity Clinics*. These will be discussed below. However, due to the nature of the analysis detailed in the method section, the hermeneutic of suspicion sections above will have covered some of the discursive material more commonly found in the discussion and so I will not needlessly reiterate them here. Consequently in the section below

I will concentrate on the wider implications of the research findings and their implications for existential-phenomenological counselling psychological practice particularly, as well as the limitations of this research, and possibilities for future directions which workers in this field might consider.

Limitations and strengths of the study, and future directions

A key element of this study, and indeed phenomenological enquiry in general, is that the participants were asked to communicate about themselves, while being aware that such communication is necessarily flawed. Butler (2005) comments in *Giving an account of oneself* that a true account is not possible as people will necessarily not have been aware during the formative period of the Self in childhood and, further, that such a Self will evolve and change – even in the process of giving the account. Additionally, language is such that there is no absolute shared meaning – both interlocutors will have different understandings of a communicative act. As she makes clear:

> [T]he "I" has no story of its own that is not also the story of a relation – or set of relations – to a set of norms. . . . The "I" is always to some extent dispossessed by the social conditions of its emergence.
>
> (Butler, 2005, p. 8)

Gadamer (2004 [1960]) suggests that this interlocution will therefore involve a fusion of horizons, and indeed in terms of the hermeneutic of description above that is what is sought. However when considering the hermeneutic of suspicion, even allowing for a degree of reflexive epoché, there will still be something of me, as a researcher and invariably as a person, which will bleed through (Langdridge, 2007; 2013). Indeed there is a further iteration in what you, the reader, make of my words here as you too will have understandings which differ from my intended communication – despite my (our) best efforts (Richards, 2011a).

Another issue with regards to receiving the intended communication is that of the medium through which such communication flows. In the case of the present research this is approximately as follows in Figure 5.1 (although this diagram does not allow for the added complexity of the group discussion with multiple participants).

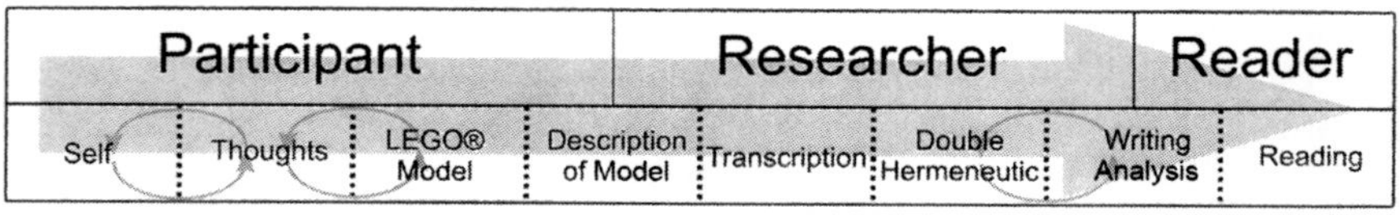

Participant				Researcher			Reader
Self	Thoughts	LEGO® Model	Description of Model	Transcription	Double Hermeneutic	Writing Analysis	Reading

Figure. 5.1 Medium of communication flow

We have dealt elsewhere with the complexities of responding to the Other and within oneself (as in the feedback loops in Figure 5.1), but here it is worth considering the actual medium – the LEGO®, the description, the writing (and the reading). The issue here is that there will necessarily be a disjoint between the mediums in what may be considered to be an expansion of Derrida (1998 [1967]) who argued against Saussure's (1916) assertion that "Language and writing are two distinct systems of signs; the second exists for the sole purpose of representing the first" (p. 45). This is poststructuralist, of course, as Derrida suggested that writing would always be a different representation of meaning than language, and indeed in the present study writing must represent the LEGO® model rather than just language per se. This is effectively insoluble, of course[1] and it is hoped that the benefits of the media outweigh the costs.

A key element of these communication problems concerns labels – not just in the sense of words – but in the literal sense of strong (restricting) signifiers – especially for sexual and gender identities and practices. As we will see below under the theme of Reference to Multiplicity or Binary Identities, many participants disliked the restrictive nature of labels, while still requiring them, and indeed fighting for them, in order to navigate the social world. To an ethical social scientist such as myself this presents a quandary. When Cee Cee says, "I want to, um and be sexually free . . . of labels, sexuality labels", how do I write about them without using words as labels? Of course in the crass sense I can refrain from using labels such as Bisexual, Gay, Lesbian, Heterosexual, etc., but in a subtle sense all writing is fixing, determining, setting down and in that sense I am concerned that I am therefore doing a disservice to the participants which might act as an ethical violation of an already marginalised group. Nonetheless the participants were fully aware of the intent of the research and that it involved writing, and so I have endeavoured to tread lightly while not asserting overmuch academy-derived power in fixing participant identities.

An interrelated area of issue is that it is difficult to find an ontological space concerned with trans people qua trans people as this study was undertaken (as it must be) within a global context of the marginalisation of trans people and adherence to cisgender norms. This is analogous to Irigaray's arguments concerning [cisgender] female subjectivity on which Spinelli (2014) comments, "Irigaray argues that female subjectivity has not, as yet, been identified because it continues to be assimilated to male subjectivity" (p. 48). I agree, and therefore would like to make the same argument here for trans and cisgender subjectivities respectively. In so long as trans people wish to 'pass' as cisgender and indeed relate their lives to those of cisgender people in terms of legal recognition, reproduction, etc., trans subjectivities will be simply a shadow of cisgender subjectivities. This is not to say that trans people should not have precisely the same things which make up cisgender subjectivities (and much else besides), but that they should be on their own terms – trans qua trans. Only at this point will research and therapy with trans people truly be *with* trans people – whether they and cisgender people live in the same way or not. Thus this global context forms a significant limitation for the study in terms of establishing a 'truth' about trans people, but perhaps is useful in finding out about trans people *now* and the *implicit relation to cisgender people*.

One element of contention in the literature which may be a result of this lack of emancipated trans subjectivities (and perhaps including an argument for such subjectivities) is that concerning autogynephilia and autoandrophilia. It is notable that none of the participants chose to reference this contentious subject. This could be because it *is* such a contentious subject, yet the participants felt free to disagree on other matters. It may be that it is more of a US phenomenon – certainly it occurs much more in US literatures and is extremely uncommon in clinical contexts in the UK (Richards & Barker, 2013). Or perhaps it is just not a useful concept for considering trans people's erotic thoughts which include themselves as sexual subjects. Indeed, Bettcher (2014) argues instead for erotic structuralism

> Which replaces an exclusively other-directed account of gendered attraction with one that includes a gendered eroticization of self as an essential component. This erotic experience of self is necessary for other-directed gendered desire, where the two are bound together and mutually informing.
> (p. 605)

Certainly this would seem to accord more with the participants' responses which included both their, and their sexual partners', genders. That trans people wish to include their and their partner's gender in their sexual expression seems trivial, and is certainly also the case for cisgender people (Attwood et al., 2013).

More prosaically in terms of limitations, as this was a qualitative study all of the usual positives and negatives associated with that (which are detailed in the method above) will apply. Most notably, given the findings associated with heterogeneity, it is likely that a different group, especially one from a markedly different cultural background, would likely have different understandings regarding sexuality and gender. Consequently, further work with explicitly chosen cultural groups may yield interesting findings. Indeed, it is tempting to consider specific demographic details beyond culture as another avenue of enquiry and again there may be interesting findings to be found. One detail which may be of note is that of genital surgical status, as sexuality can change after surgery (Coleman & Bockting, 1989; Lawrence, 2005; Rowniak & Chesla, 2013). However trans communities, especially online ones, are becoming ever more heterogeneous – with more people becoming non-operative rather than simply pre-or post-operative and so researchers should exercise caution in creating artificial divisions where they do not exist, especially as we move into a more complex (internet connected) world. As ever, close attention to the research question and the appropriate demographic to that will be key. In the current study, for example, consideration was given as to whether to have only a group of trans men or trans women or non-binary trans people. A single group may indeed have led to interesting participant responses, however, given the complexity and heterogeneity of the responses regarding gender, what this would actually mean would be difficult to ascertain. Indeed it may actually act as a false researcher imposition on the responses rather than a reasonable structural research procedure. Certainly the cross–trans themes elicited here could not be recognised if such a division were to be put in place.

It was, in fact, one of the key methodological considerations underlying this research that researcher impact be minimised. For example, in order to minimise researcher impact upon the participants' explanations and discussion it was decided after the pilot to minimise researcher 'presence' in this work. Consequently, further work (whether with a similar or different cultural range from the present study) in which the participant responses are more closely interrogated at the time may yield fruitful findings – although this will, of course, mean more researcher 'presence' which will likely affect the explanations for both good and ill, and the ethics of this should naturally be considered carefully in light of the ethical considerations detailed above. Indeed, even in the current study, the use of interjections such as "great" by the researcher as encouragement may have still been taken as affirmation from a position of power by participants, and could usefully be considered in future research.

There was an ethical tension also in representing the humanity of the participants given that they were anonymised. Each participant chose their pseudonym in order to mitigate this to some extent, and my hope is that there has not been too much over-theorisation or especially theoretical imposition as can too often be found in work which treats participants words and identities as just things – indeed, one might argue, treats participants as just things, because this would be entirely unethical (c.f. Pratchett, 1998).

I am hopeful, however, that a strength of this research is the ethical stance which was taken. It seems apposite, therefore to cede the floor to one of the participants, Mr Fox, for the last word on this:

> "I was really sort of surprised, and I really enjoyed the kind of *richness* that came out of people's different models and the way that they talked about it and stuff so I thought that was that was quite a, kind of, *useful*, um kind of tool really. . . . There's something about [the research which is] very much kind of, human, humanising process. And I think, I think when I think about how trans people are represented in terms of our sexuality we're very, very *de*humanised."

Themes

Barriers

One of the main themes found was that of barriers – both with regards to society and concerning transitioning. This theme intersected with the theme of *Gender Identity Clinics* in that the clinics were sometimes seen as a barrier to transitioning and consequently matters pertaining to them will be discussed below in the relevant section.

One of the key elements concerning barriers was that of relating to others in an authentic manner and of the difficulties associated with that. For some participants this was mediated by having a congruent body though transition and for others this was about society having a greater and more nuanced understanding of the diversity of trans identities. In both cases it is about not being seen as who one is. This can also be extended to not seeing *oneself* as who one is due to the disjoint between identity and gender(ed body, expression, and so on). Of course folded up in this is sexuality, which is both implicit and permeating as Merleau-Ponty would have it (Merleau-Ponty, 1996 [1945]), and the literal, explicit (in both senses of the word) act of fucking.

In considering barriers then, we must consider intersubjectivity and the overcoming of such barriers, for such intersubjectivity might be between two individuals or within a single being. Within a single being it can concern relating either over long spans of time (how to I relate to my younger or older selves) or more recently (I want the cake, but don't allow myself). In addition, we might consider ideas within our self which are not fully in consciousness but which we nonetheless relate to: Why am I singing this song now? Why was I so mean to my friend on the phone? If sexuality does indeed permeate our selves like an atmosphere, especially if it does indeed permeate intersubjectivity, it should permeate such self–self encounters also. Indeed it may permeate whether we see our full selves as selves or as objects, as in Cooper's (2003) I-I or I-Me relating.

Thus gender/sexual relating interacts in complex ways, both within the conceptual limits of the person's body, and also in the wider sense in which gender and sexuality permeate the person's self, and on to society. In this vein Gagne & Tewksbury (2002) suggest the idea of "gendered sexualities" which are "The ways in which individual and societal constructions of gender overlay and intermingle with sexual behaviours, ideations, attitudes, identities, and experiences" (p. 4), however this does not include the internal interactions between gender and sexuality, the biological substrates, and the way body and self are situated within society (and the epistemic feedback of this situation). A diagram in Figure 5.2 may assist (although please assume the drawn boundaries are fuzzy).

We can see here that the barriers that trans people feel towards intersubjective authentic relating may be from others (or to others) or within one's self in various ways, and as such may form part of the clinical encounter which considers gendered and sexual intersubjectivity(ies). Consequently when Manafi (2014) suggests that "Being sexual is an embodied interrelational engagement" (p. xi), there may be a single embodiment (within oneself), or two, or many (indeed there may be none in the traditional sense if one allows virtual embodiment online).

In terms of addressing such barriers within counselling psychological practice, it may be useful to establish the location and type of such barriers: Are they within the client as a sort of internalised transphobia where the trans self is split off? Or are they from society? Or towards society as a means of keeping safe? As ever, a phenomenological explanation and getting alongside the client will

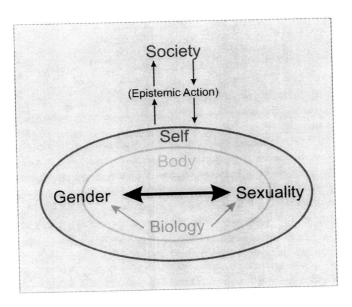

Figure 5.2 Sexuality and gender in body and society

be useful. I would also suggest (following Langdridge, 2014) that being affirmative of trans identities in general may be useful to mitigate against some of the
discourses against Gender and Sexual Diverse (GSD) people's lives.

Time

One of the key themes which intersects with *Barriers* is that of *Time*, as naturally
the formation and overcoming of barriers will be situated within time. Indeed (as
we change levels of analysis) existentially it may be said that Being is being in time,
or indeed that Being *is* time (Heidegger, 2008 [1962]) as both our prereflective and
reflective consciousness is thrown into a world where we exist towards death. Certainly, the sense of becoming we all experience is writ large in trans people's lives
when transitioning. But as stated above, this becoming will be inflected by both
past and future and should not be seen as a uni-directional becoming (or indeed
a trans-specific state of affairs as there are many different forms of transition in all
people's lives). In the simple sense, such becoming will reflect the greater congru-
ence trans people feel after transition, and so the greater possibilities for sexuality
and sexual expression. As Schilt & Windsor (2014) note, for example:

> Trans men's transformed gendered embodiment can result in a greater sense
> of continuity between their bodies, their personal gender identity, and their
> social gender (how they are seen by others).
>
> (p. 744)

This reflects the efficacy of interventions for trans people (Gijs & Brewaeys, 2007; Ruppin & Pfafflin, 2015), but does not situate such interventions fully within the complex flow of prereflective understanding and reflective understanding that being-in-the-world invites. Indeed it is trite to suggest that an embodied sexuality may be improved if a congruent body is available, but it is also true to say that a new understanding may inflect a memory of a previously incongruent body such that it is reconstrued. Further, in being towards death, time inflects understandings of embodiment and sexuality – not just directly in the sense of 'time running out' and 'waiting' as some participants explained, but also in less apparently chronological concerns such as the type of sexual expression available, as it is what is available *now* – with understandings drawn from the past, thoughts of what may be thought and felt in the future, and a consideration that such an opportunity may or may not be available in the time to come.

In this way we may see embodiment as situated within time, indeed as constituted of time. Further intersubjectivity – indeed what I have characterised above as the interobjective gaze of the Other – capturing an Other happens in a moment, but a moment in time. If one is to agree with Sartre (2003 [1943]) who posits that sexuality is where one acquires and is acquired by the Other, that process must be one of intentionality where the (likely prereflective) sexuality of a person is expressed through the ready-to-hand body, or between individuals in some other way, in an evolving process in time in which both becoming beings (be)come together.[2]

Another way to contextualise this is in a consideration of the different forms of time posited by Ricoeur (1984; 1985; 1988): cosmological time (time in the vast stretches in which the universe operates), phenomenological time (our, far briefer, experienced time), and historical time (in some sense the bridge between the two in which events are marked and recalled or considered for the future). As seen above, trans community themes of previous policy and practice by GICs, for example, may fall into historical time, which inflects the phenomenological time which trans people currently experience.

Time then, is a theme which resonates with many trans people as considerations of past (both phenomenological and historical) and future inflect the present. For counselling psychologists it can be tempting to consider the past in terms of whether physical alterations have been undertaken and, while this may be a question to be considered, it is only a small part of the meaning of time for trans people. Similarly, future wishes may again be brought into the therapy room – not uncommonly whether to transition or not, and if so, how? (Richards & Barker, 2013). But again this is only a part of the meaning of time. While perhaps not explicitly considering all of the above with all trans clients, it may be useful to consider how such philosophies and understandings may affect this client work.

Reference to multiplicity or binary identities

Both binary and multiple identities figured largely in the participant's responses. Both discourses were readily available, with several participants resisting binary identities, quite often as being societally normative constructions. However, some participants, notably Mr Fox, also resisted the notion of multiplicity (in the form of queer) specifically as it pertained to him. Indeed the notion of multiplicity itself had varying meanings, being both something fluid and changing and also something with discrete yet multiple categories. These elements pertained both to sexuality and gender and, again, sexuality and gender intertwined in complex ways so as to not be wholly distinguishable from one another, yet at the same time often being linguistically discrete. An exception to this was the term *queer*, which was used, as it often is, to trouble the notion of a split between gender and sexuality – and indeed queer theory was cited, which troubles the notion of ontological splits in any field (Barker, Richards, Bowes-Catton & Gupta, 2009).

Intersecting with the theme of *Barriers* and *Time* above, binaries were considered in both the sense of overcoming a discrete barrier (across time) and also in moving in a more fluid way within and between different identities and practices. Consequently, for some participants, binary conceptions of sexuality and gender were coherent and authentic ways of expressing themselves in the world – for example as a man who is attracted to other men and their identity as being gay, or as a woman who is attracted to men and their identity as being heterosexual. However, other participants used discrete terms for entities associated with sexuality and of gender because non-discrete terms were not available in English, while feeling this fell short of their intended communication. In this way a disjoint was formed between the 'text' of the LEGO® model and the conversion into English for the explanation. Butler (1999; 2005) speaks to this when she suggests that language breaks down when endeavouring to address such identities and practices, as language is structurally more discrete and contiguous than such fluidity and complexity warrants. This is, in a sense, similar to that which we have noted above with regard to Derrida (1998 [1967]) in that it is a poststructuralist position in which experience and language are decoupled which makes the task of research in this field difficult without doing a disservice to those participants for whom the language I am using is insufficient. I do not, of course, wish to be the 'society' which some participants felt was constraining their expression in this way.

Notwithstanding this, it is evident that some participants rear-grounded their fluid identities on a day-to-day basis, and especially when engaging with the GICs, in order to be comprehensible to their interlocutors and so navigate the social world without undue difficulty. In this way the Other can be seen to be acquiring and socially constructing some more fluid trans participants through the (lack of) available discourse. Indeed even those trans participants with binary identities often felt constrained by the language available for their explanations as the binaries available did not always encompass trans experience – perhaps because some binaries have a non-binary element in the sense of moving between two (binary) nodes. This paradoxical engagement with language and labelling concerning sex and gender in particular was noted several times and is of particular relevance for counselling psychologists engaging with trans clients as language may not be a fully effective medium for such engagement. For example, a client who says that they are heterosexual might have a great deal more meaning within that label than at first may be apparent.

Having said this, labels are, as we have seen, politically necessary. The arguments made above concerning the ethical difficulties of deconstructing a client's stated identity into a multiple, fluid, entity will not needlessly be repeated here, but this quote from Crabtree (2009) speaks eloquently:

> An over emphasis on the fluidity and plasticity of our sexual experiences may lead to a therapeutic practice which is out of touch with the client's lived experience of their sexual attractions and sexual identity.
>
> (p. 258)

This is pertinent because cisgender and heteronormative clients seldom experience such deconstruction of identity, even if it is deemed to be philosophically valid (which I am unsure of). Consequently we have another paradox: Clients may both have a label which they use and which they disagree with, and relatedly counselling psychologists may wish to consider the multiplicity of meaning with a binary frame. An example of this might be found with cisgender people where it is commonly accepted that there are men and that there are women: But it is also understood that there are no psychological categories in which these entities are discrete. Indeed those people who have more flexibility (within the extant binary societal frame) to undertake masculine and feminine tasks and thought process are psychologically healthier (Bem & Lenney, 1976). Another example would be a man who has sex with other men and for whom we might use the sexual health term *MSM*, but who does not accept the label gay because he does not identify as such. As Hicks & Milton (2010) note:

> What does knowing someone's sexual *identity*[3] actually tell us? The answer is arguably nothing. Knowing an individual's sexual identity does not automatically convey any information regarding a person's sexual behaviours or attractions, rather it might simply be a sign of a current identification with a particular social grouping.
>
> (p. 261)

Thus a split between practice and identity can be a useful frame for viewing such fluidity and fixity (cf. Richards & Barker, 2013; 2015) which does not needlessly impose a philosophy of reduction onto the client's worlding.

Gender Identity Clinics

The last major theme which arose was *Gender Identity Clinics*. It is notable that this theme arose at all considering that the research question posed concerned the participants' sexuality and did not mention GICs. Consequently one of the first queries regarding this theme is why *did* it arise at all? A possible answer to this requires a little explanation, so I beg your forbearance for a paragraph or two.

What I endeavoured to do in this monograph, indeed what I imagine most phenomenologists try to do in their work, is to get to the heart of the participant's worlding, to hear how things are *for them*. Theirs (indeed everyone's) worlding will necessarily be an intersubjective worlding, which will draw on available discourses as a means of both construction and communication (Butler, 2005). Although aware of this intersubjectivity, my hope (my fantasy?) is that the participants' own creative reality could be touched in some way without undue interference from me, that my part in the intersubjectivity would be as passive as possible. (If the reader will forgive a metaphor) I hope the participants felt their communication was as free as if they were in an area, perhaps a field, in which they could roam as they chose, to point out their privileges and their passions, the boundaries and the freedoms which form their world. I imagine a field on the moon so there is even more freedom of travel away up and gently down again too. Of course there are some constraints in such a field, but freedom is inherent in the domain. It seems however, that much discourse – even that acquired phenomenologically – is something more akin to a road network – still with a good deal of freedom, but constrained too – often within certain boundaries of class, culture, language, the wish to please the researcher, and the such.

Trans, however, seems sometimes to be more akin to a railway leading always back to the GICs – the rails laid together by clinicians[4] who circumscribe lived experience through protocols (RCP, 2013; WPATH, 2011) and by the participant-patients who, in acceding or resisting these, are constructed by that discourse. This is why studies on such things as trans people's partners so often refer to the GICs (Sanger, 2010) and why studies on bodily aesthetics do also (Davy, 2008). To some extent this was the purpose of use of LEGO® in the current study – to try to circumnavigate these accreted scripts, and yet the wider discourse pertaining to the gender clinics seems so central to the realities of many trans people that it will out regardless – it will inflect, inform, indeed construct trans people's worlding – including their gender and sexuality.

How could it not we may ask? A protocol which is wary of fetishism on the grounds that it is likely to lead to regret after surgical interventions will likely inform practice in this area (Barrett, 2007), as is one which examines penis and/or vagina intercourse on the grounds that people using their penis or vagina may regret losing them (ibid). New ways of being intimate must be discussed (Ettner, Monstrey & Eyler, 2007), as must fertility and the development of secondary sexual characteristics (Richards & Seal, 2014) – all in order that a trans person can have their embodied self realised. In many cases these discussions literally take years. How could this not so often create an overarching discourse inflecting many trans people's (sexual) worlding?

This, I believe, is why the theme of the GICs was so pertinent, and perhaps especially so in the group discussion. Discussions among trans people, both online and face-to-face, about clinics and clinical protocols are commonplace and therefore will have been a familiar discourse to many participants. Perhaps this is why there was less (although not none) consideration given to the GICs in the model discussions as the models had performed their job of avoiding accreted scripts. These group discourses, both in this research and elsewhere, will inform and construct personal, internal, trans discourses also and it may be argued are also therefore constitutive. We can imagine that trans people who have not had to attend a clinical setting to access treatments may nonetheless have a view of clinical settings, for example. Thus the GICs are a common constituent factor in many trans people's worlding, even if they were not intended to be. Indeed such constitution may act as a barrier in people's lives – both with regards to the reality of their encounters with the clinics and also intrapsychically. This will occur in time as it inflects the experience of people who attend the clinics both before and after engagement, and also within discussion groups on and off line – so inflecting the worlding of trans people who have not attended such clinics.

This anger and distrust of the GICs is clearly a difficult issue which needs addressing (and which is being so). Indeed, it should be noted that participants will be aware of my position within the GICs and some of the purpose of their discourse may be in communicating their message back, both through the formal research process and possibly in the hope that I will carry the discourse with me personally. This is not a forlorn hope, as I explicitly stated I will carry the findings back to the GICs, and I cannot but be inflected and impacted through undertaking the research. Hopefully in this way participants can feel that I (and by extension others) have got 'alongside' them rather than being in some way adversarial. Indeed, an extension of this approach may be a key means of addressing the anger and distrust of GICs mentioned above – it may be useful for clinical protocols too to borrow from counselling psychological and existential philosophies and to recommend that an attempt is made to get 'alongside' the client through a phenomenological investigation of their worlding. Once a full(er) picture has been sketched out, assistance may be offered which is apposite *for that client* and which includes both freedom and responsibility. In this way the protocol-driven procrustean approach, which many participants felt was unhelpful as it did not reflect their own reality, may be changed instead to the creation of a safe space in which clients can make a 'leap to faith' – in this case the faith being their own biopsychosociospiritual authenticity regarding sexuality, gender, and the worlding which is permeated by these.

Implications for practice

While these findings cannot be said to be universal or true in all times and all places as, of course, they will be peculiar to this group, there is some degree of generalisability for similar groups in that such themes may be regarded as philosophically likely to apply to other trans people also. The research is also 'generalisable' in the sense that it is factually true, almost tautologically so, that *some* trans people do these things, i.e. of the general body of trans people some do these things. This may seem trivial, however, it allows us to rebut universalisation from research and theory which suggests that all (or none) do such things. Thus this research rebuts the assertion that all trans people are heterosexual in their identified gender, for example.

The key implication for practice derived from this research therefore is arguably that counselling psychologists should attend to the lived experience of their clients. Again, this may seem so trivial as to be trite, given this stance is so central to counselling psychological practice (Woolfe, Dryden & Strawbridge, 2003), however, this research has at least reiterated this most important point which occasionally gets forgotten when counselling psychologists endeavour to work in reductionist fields such as the NHS and funded research (Clark & Loewenthal, 2015) and indeed may be of use to other professions also. As part of this attending to the client's lived experience there will necessarily be the use of extreme caution in the application of theory as this has not always well served non-heterosexual and non-cisgender clients (cf. Judd & Milton, 2001). As one of the participants, Cee Cee, noted:

> "The worst thing is that a lot of practitioners are not *aware*, of, of these [heteronormative] biases that they're bringing into their assessments and work that you're doing just now, us talking is really important that they get that."

Instead, the basis of phenomenological, and indeed existential-phenomenological, practice should be attended to – that of being with the client and exploring their world in a supportive manner.

Of course this does not mean that clients should not be challenged. Indeed clients often come to therapy for one of two reasons – they can't fully see what their difficulty is and would like assistance uncovering it, or they know what their difficulty is but don't feel able to do anything about it (whether in terms of acceptance or change). Either of these may involve challenge, regarding both acting in the world and acting intrapsychically. One of the key issues commonly requiring such challenge with regard to both sexuality and gender is that of prejudice (Richards & Barker, 2015). Such prejudice may come from external sources and so cause marginalisation stress, but may also come from internal sources and so be internalised *phobia – be it trans-, homo-, bi-, etc. Judd & Milton (2001) comment that:

> With its attentiveness to issues such as relatedness, personal responsibility, choice and meaninglessness, the existential-phenomenological paradigm provides trainees (and training providers) with a theoretical and therapeutic approach which is equipped to challenge sedimented, [trans- and][5] homo-negative biases and assumptions which may be maintained, minimised, silenced or simply ignored through other models of therapy.
>
> (p. 7)

I quite agree. One key means of doing this is recognising the latitude which is available within people's worldviews and moving from there: If it is ok to be trans for other people why not for you (the client)?; Where is the line between spicy sex and unacceptable BDSM? Indeed, crucially, what does it *mean* to be trans and gay, or trans and heterosexual? What does it mean for each individual client to be these things? In this way sedimented beliefs may be able to be loosened through supportive enquiry and horizontalisation rather than crass reductionism.

This is not to say that counselling psychologists should utilise this theory in an unconsidered manner either. As seen throughout the analysis above, both labels and complexity should be allowed. Indeed, given that trans and non-heterosexual people often have to defend their identities due to these identities not being given to them by society at birth, extra care should be taken not to reiterate such structural oppression though doubting the label, or indeed questioning its veracity – Milton (2005): "As Frankl and others highlight the ignoring of identity can be as difficult personally and politically powerful as the enforcement of another identity" (p. 247). This does create a challenge for ethical counselling psychologists who wish to investigate sexuality and gender, and perhaps will be especially so for those clients who have non-binary or genderqueer identities as these naturally invite a consideration of fluidity and the inappropriateness of labels. Indeed as these identities are only recently emerging into wider public discourse, labels themselves are likely to change and counselling psychologists should be wary of appearing to misunderstand such identities through correlating a change of label with an instability of identity – although again without throwing out the baby of enquiry with the bathwater of erroneous theory.

This use of a wider frame of phenomenology, and perhaps also existential-phenomenological practice, instead of strict theory-driven practice (as in psychoanalysis and some other modalities), may also address the ethical practice and research quandary over who controls trans people's stories. As seen with the autogynephilia debates detailed in the literature review, the appropriation of trans narratives and lives to buttress theory has a long and troubling history (cf. Richards, Barker, Lenihan & Iantaffi, 2014). Indeed this history continues to impact therapy as trans people who are aware of these debates often instinctively distrust clinicians whom they assume will misinterpret their narratives though this (false) theoretical lens or, it is feared, may appropriate the narrative to build or adapt a theoretical lens. Instead, given the complexity we have seen in this analysis, only the most light touch theory should be used and a frame consisting of ethical practice alongside the client would seem far more appropriate.

Lastly, the matters we have considered above in relation to trans people, including how bodies, gender, and sexuality inflect and inform one another, should also be considered for cisgender people. Cisgender people will almost invariably not have considered their gender in the depth that a trans client will and, if they state they are heterosexual, may not have considered their sexuality either and so may give a less reflective account of themselves. This means that cisgender clients may not have mapped out areas of disjoint and so be straining to fill them in order to fit with an assumed universal norm of a given gender and sexuality which is apocryphal. For example, a cisgender man may be concerned about his penis and what it means to be a man – and much can be learned here in considering trans male experience. Erectile dysfunction and various forms of sex may be usefully explored – again drawing on trans women's experience. These parallels may not be explicit, of course, as some cisgender people resent comparison to trans people, but nonetheless useful consideration can be undertaken which informs both trans and cisgender people.

Another useful element to take from the trans research detailed here which may be applied in counselling psychological work with cisgender people is that of labels and the complexity and fluidity within them. Cisgender people have a number of labels which are used, and indeed in some cases have labels which are so prevalent as to be effectively invisible (for example *cisgender*). These labels will contain within them significant fluidity and diversity in both identity and practice, and consequently counselling psychologists may do well to explore the fluidity without necessarily challenging the veracity of the cisgender client's labels.

Summary of recommendations for counselling psychological practice

- Be aware of the diversity of trans experience.
- Be aware that people may be both binary and non-binary.
- Refrain from inserting trans and non-binary people into either reductionist or postmodernist philosophical frameworks in a procrustean manner.
- Consider allowing ethics to trump philosophy when in a therapeutic quandary.
- Consider how findings concerning authenticity and the considered life in trans experience may also be of use with cisgender clients' considerations of sexuality and gender.

Conclusion

The trans people in this study were heterogeneous but, as seen above, shared several common concerns – most pertinently those of being constrained and misunderstood, both in regards to the complexity of their identities and practices concerning sexuality and gender, and in regards to the simplicity of them. Indeed the very notions of sexuality and gender as discrete categories and their intersections with wider identity became troubled. Consequently any overriding theory presented here would be suspect and indeed may be unethical in that it would seek to constrain the participants' contributions which spoke to both identity as a felt concrete entity and a complexity within that. Therefore only such wider themes as are detailed above, and the overarching theme of the necessity of recognising both identity and fluidity as ontologically non-conflictual entities are given here. To reiterate, this is not to say that all trans people have a fluid identity, but that a variety of meanings can be found within any given identity *which is nonetheless valid and true as a discreet identity*. In this way we may see trans people's sexuality as both postmodern and reductionist. Therefore the diagnostic terms we referred to at the beginning of this monograph appear to be perhaps somewhat philosophically flawed in that, as entities designed to demarcate strict boundaries, they lack the power to fully encompass fluidity, multiplicity, and the complex relationship to time seen here, as well as the discrete reductionist categories and process of labelling they sit within.

Trans people then, are identifying and practicing a number of different genders and sexualities and these are, of course, all valid. These things inflect and inform more widely – both within the person (including how they relate to themselves) and also, of course, in relation to others in the world. These others will, in a sort of epistemic feedback loop, naturally inflect, and indeed constitute, the trans person themselves – just as the trans person is inflecting and constituting the other. Thus for a counselling psychologist concerned with intersubjective relating, the 'sexuality' we are considering here is not so much fucking as Being, which is, of course, a being-in-the-world (with others including ourselves). It would be perverse for our practice to attempt to subvert this into a reductionist theory-driven notion of pure complexity or fluidity – or indeed to concretise identity alone. Consequently this research finds that for a counselling psychologist to act ethically a paradox may have to be held.

So be it.

Notes

1 Alas, I was not allowed to defend the thesis this monograph is based upon by means of a LEGO® model. . . . Viva parvis plasticus lateres similiter imperantur inter profeci, densis, if you will. . . . Ahem.
2 Please insert your own pun as you feel appropriate.
3 Italics my own.
4 Who may be trans of course.
5 My own insertion.

References

Acton, H. (2010). I am what I am: Existentialism and homosexuality. *Existential Analysis, 21* (2), 351–364.

American Psychiatric Association (APA). (1980). *Diagnostic and statistical manual of mental disorders III*. Washington, DC: American Psychiatric Association.

American Psychiatric Association (APA). (2013a). *Diagnostic and statistical manual of mental disorders 5*. Washington, DC: American Psychiatric Association.

American Psychiatric Association (APA). (2013b). *Gender dysphoria*. Washington, DC: American Psychiatric Association.

Atnas, C., Milton, M., & Archer, S. (2015). Making the decision to change – the experiences of trans men. *Counselling Psychology Review, 30* (1), 33–42.

Attwood, F., Bale, C., Barker, M., Albury, K., Angel, K., Bragg, S., Brooks-Gordon, B., Chronaki, D., Duschinsky, R., Egan, R. D., Gill, R., Hammond, N., Hancock, J., Hoggart, L., Hubbard, P., Kermode, J., Lee, J., Lewis, R., McGeeney, E., McKee, A., Mercer, J., Klein, M., das Nair, R., Renold, E., Richards, C., Ringrose, J., Roen, K., Smith, C., Tiefer, L., Tsaliki, L., van Zoonen. L., & Weitzer, R. (2013). *The sexualisation report*. Milton Keynes: The Open University.

Auer, M. K., Fuss, J., Hohne, N., Stalla, G. K., & Sievers, C. (2014). Transgender transitioning and change of self-reported sexual orientation. *PLoS One, 9* (10), e110016. doi: 10.1371/journal.pone.0110016

Ault, A., & Brzuzy, S. (2009). Removing gender identity disorder from the diagnostic and statistical manual of mental disorders: A call for action. *Social Work, 54* (2), 187–189.

Bailey, J. M. (2003). *The man who would be queen: The science of gender-bending and transsexualism*. Washington, DC: Joseph Henry Press.

Bao, A-M., & Swaab, D. F. (2011). Sexual differentiation of the human brain: Relation to gender identity, sexual orientation and neuropsychiatric disorders. *Frontiers in Neuroendocrinology, 32*, 214–226.

Barker, M. (2006). Sexual self-disclosure and outness in academia and the clinic. *Lesbian & Gay Psychology Review, 7*(3), 292–296.

Barker, M., Bowes-Catton, H., Iantaffi, A., Cassidy, A., & Brewer, L. (2008). British bisexuality: A snapshot of bisexual identities in the UK. *Journal of Bisexuality, 8*, 141–162.

Barker, M., Richards, C., & Bowes-Catton, H. (2012). Visualising experience: Using creative research methods with members of sexual communities. In C. Phellas (Ed.), *Researching non-heterosexual sexualities* (pp. 57–79). Farnham: Ashgate.

Barker, M., Richards, C., Bowes-Catton, H., & Gupta, C. (2009). 'All the world is queer save thee and me . . .'": Defining queer and bi at a Critical Sexology seminar. *Journal of Bisexuality, 9*, 363–379.

Barrett, J. (Ed.). (2007). *Transsexual and other disorders of gender identity*. Oxford: Radcliffe.

Basch, C. E. (1987). Focus group interviews: An underutilized technique for improving theory and practice in health education. *Health Education Quarterly, 14*, 411–448.

Beard, G. M. (1886). *Sexual neurasthenia (nervous exhaustion): Its hygiene, cases symptoms and treatment*. New York: NY EB Treat.

Bem, S. L., & Lenney, E. (1976). Sex typing and the avoidance of cross-sex behavior. *Journal of Personality and Social Psychology, 33* (1), 48.

Benjamin, H. (1966). *The transsexual phenomenon*. New York: The Julian Press, Inc.

Benson, K. E. (2013). Seeking support: Transgender client experiences with mental health services. *Journal of Feminist Family Therapy, 25* (1), 17–40.

Bentall, R. P. (2003). *Madness explained*. London: Penguin.

Bergman, S. B. (2009). *The nearest exit may be behind you*. Vancouver: Arsenal Pulp Press.

Bettcher, T. M. (2014). When selves have sex: What the phenomenology of trans sexuality can teach about sexual orientation. *Journal of Homosexuality, 61* (5), 605–620.

Blanchard, R. (1989). The concept of autogynephilia and the typology of male gender dysphoria. *Journal of Nervous and Mental Diseases, 177*, 616–623.

Blanchard, R. (1991). Clinical observations and systematic studies of autogynephilia. *Journal of Sex and Marital Therapy, 17* (4), 235–251.

Bockting, W. O. (2008). Psychotherapy and the real-life experience: From gender dichotomy to gender diversity. *Sexologies, 17* (4), 211–224.

Bockting, W. O., Benner, A., & Coleman, E. (2009). Gay and bisexual identity development among female-to-male transsexuals in North America: Emergence of a transgender sexuality. *Archives of Sexual Behavior, 38* (5), 688–701.

Bockting, W. O., & Coleman, E. (2007). Developmental stages of the transgender coming out process: Toward an integrated identity. In R. Ettner, S. Monstrey, & A. E. Eyler (Eds.), *Principles of transgender medicine and surgery* (pp. 185–208). New York: The Haworth Press.

Bockting, W. O., & Ehrbar, R. D. (2006). Commentary: Gender variance, dissonance, or identity disorder? *Journal of Psychology & Human Sexuality, 17* (3–4), 125–134.

Bockting, W. O., Rosser, B. R., & Coleman, E. (2000). Transgender HIV prevention: A model education workshop. *Journal of the Gay and Lesbian Medical Association, 4* (4), 175–183.

Bornstein, K. (1994). *Gender outlaw*. London: Routledge.

Bornstein, K. (2012). *A queer and pleasant danger: A memoir*. Boston, MA: Beacon Press Books.

Bornstein, K., & Bergman, S. B. (Eds.). (2010). *Gender outlaws: The next generation*. New York, NY: Avalon Publishing Group.

Bouman, W. P., Richards, C., Whitcomb, G., de Vries, A., & Kreukels, B. (in prep). *United Kingdom field test of the proposed Gender Incongruence diagnosis in the International Classification of Diseases Version 10*. Geneva: WHO.

Bowes-Catton, H., Barker, M., & Richards, C. (2011). 'I didn't know that I could feel this relaxed in my body': Using visual methods to research bisexual people's embodied experiences of identity and space. In P. Reavey (Ed.), *Visual psychologies: Using and interpreting images in qualitative research* (pp. 255–270). London: Routledge.

Boylan, J. F. (2003). *She's not there: A life in two genders*. New York: Broadway Books.

BPS (British Psychological Society). [Cranbourne, M., Draysey, D., Finnigan, J., Gilbert, K., Golsworthy, R., Hall, A., Hammersley, D., Moon, L., Richards, G., Walsh, Y., & Van Scoyoc, S.]. (2004). *Division of counselling psychology: Professional practice statement*. Leicester: British Psychological Society.

BPS (British Psychological Society). [Authors unlisted]. (2009). *Code of ethics and conduct*. Leicester: British Psychological Society.

BPS (British Psychological Society). [Oates, J., Coulthard, L. M., Dockrell, J., Stone, J., Foreman, N., Alderson, P., Velmans, M., Clifton, P., Kwiatkowski, R., Locke, A., Bucks, R., Macguire, N., Grant, C.]. (2010). *Code of human research ethics*. Leicester: British Psychological Society.

BPS (British Psychological Society). [Shaw, L., Butler, C., Langdridge, D., Gibson, S., Barker, M., Lenihan, P., Nair, R., Monson, J., & Richards, C.]. (2012). *Guidelines for psychologists working therapeutically with sexual minority clients*. London: British Psychological Society.

Buber, M. (1958). *I and thou* (2nd ed.) [Trans R .G. Smith]. London: Continuum.

Bullough, V., & Bullough, B. (1977). *Sin, sickness, and sanity: A history of sexual attitudes*. New York: New American Library.

Butler, J. (1988). Performative acts and gender constitution: An essay in phenomenology and feminist theory. *Theatre Journal, 40* (4), 519–531.

Butler, J. (1999). *Gender trouble*. New York: Routledge.

Butler, J. (2005). *Giving an account of oneself*. New York: Fordham University Press.

Cantarella, E. (1992). *Bisexuality in the ancient world* [Trans C. Ó. Cuilleanáin]. New Haven: Yale University Press.

Carew, L. (2009). Does theoretical background influence therapists' attitudes to therapist self-disclosure? A qualitative study. *Counselling and Psychotherapy Research, 9* (4), 266–272.

Carrigan, M. (2015). Asexuality. In C. Richards & M. J. Barker (Eds.), *The Palgrave handbook of sexuality and gender* (pp. 7–23). Basingstoke: Palgrave-Macmillan.

Cerwenka, S., Nieder, T. O., Cohen-Kettenis, P., de Cuypere, G., Haraldsen, I., & Richter-Appelt, H. (2014). *Sexual Health of Individuals with Gender Dysphoria – Findings from the ENIGI Study*. Paper presented at the 23rd Biennial International Symposium of the World Professional Association for Transgender Health entitled 'Transgender Health from Global Perspectives', Bangkok, TH, 14–18.2.2014.

Chandler, V. L., Eggleston, W. B., & Dorweiler, J. E. (2000). Paramutation in maize. *Plant Molecular Biology, 43* (2–3), 121–145.

Chiland, C. (2005). *Exploring transsexualism* [Trans D. Alcorn]. London: H. Karnac (Books) Ltd.

Chung, M. C. (1994). An outline of an existential understanding of sexual abuse. *Journal of the Society for Existential Analysis, 5*, 113–120.

Chung, W. C. J., De Vries, G. J., & Swaab, D. F. (2002). Sexual differentiation of the bed nucleus of the stria terminalis in humans may extend into adulthood. *The Journal of Neuroscience, 22* (3), 1027–1033.

Clarke, C. (2011). Barebacking and being, passion and paradox: Existentially confronting sex and mortality. *Existential Analysis, 22* (2), 244–254.

Clark, D., & Loewenthal, D. (2015). Counselling Psychology. *In The Palgrave Handbook of the Psychology of Sexuality and Gender* (pp. 280–299). Palgrave Macmillan UK.

Clarkson, N. L. (2008). Trans victims, trans zealots: A critique of Dreger's history of the Bailey controversy. *Archives of Sexual Behavior, 37* (3), 441–443.

Clements, K., Kitano, K., & Wilkinson, W. (1997). The HIV prevention and health service needs of the transgender community in San Francisco: Results from eleven focus groups. San Francisco: San Francisco Department of Public Health, AIDS Office.

Clements-Nolle, K., Marx, R., Guzman, R., Ikeda, S., & Katz, M. (2001). HIV prevalence, risk behaviors, health care use, and mental health status of transgender persons: Implications for public health intervention. *American Journal of Public Health, 91*, 915–921.

Cohn, H. W. (2014 [1997]). Being-in-the-world sexually. In M. Milton (Ed.), *Sexuality: Existential perspectives* (pp. 63–75). Ross-on-Wye: PCCS Books.

Cole, C. M., O'Boyle, M., Emory, L. E., & Meyer III, W. J. (1997). Comorbidity of gender dysphoria and other major psychiatric diagnoses. *Archives of Sexual Behavior, 26* (1), 13–26.

Coleman, E., & Bockting, W. O. (1989). 'Heterosexual' prior to sex reassignment-'homosexual' afterwards: A case study of a female-to-male transsexual. *Journal of Psychology & Human Sexuality, 1* (2), 69–82.

Coleman, E., Colgan, P., & Gooren, L. (1992). Male cross-gender behavior in Myanmar (Burma): A description of the Acault. *Archives of Sex Behavior, 21* (3), 313–321.

Colizzi, M., Costa, R., & Todarello, O. (2014). Transsexual patients' psychiatric comorbidity and positive effect of cross-sex hormonal treatment on mental health: Results from a longitudinal study. *Psychoneuroendocrinology, 39* (1), 65–73.

Coolican, H. (1994). *Research methods and statistics in psychology.* London: Hodder and Stoughton.

Cooper, M. (2003). 'I-I' and 'I-Me': Transposing Buber's interpersonal attitudes to the intra-personal plane. *Journal of Constructivist Psychology, 16* (2), 131–153.

Cossey, C. (1992). *My story.* Winchester: Faber and Faber, Inc.

Cowell, R. (1954). *Roberta Cowell's story: An autobiography.* New York: British Book Centre, Inc.

Cox, G. (2009). How to be an existentialist: Or how to get real, get a grip and stop making excuses. London: Continuum.

Crabtree, C. (2009). Rethinking sexual identity. *Existential Analysis, 20* (2), 248–261.

Crawford, L. C. (2014). Derivative plumbing: Redesigning washrooms, bodies, and trans affects in ds+ r's Brasserie. *Journal of Homosexuality, 61* (5), 621–635.

Crown, S. (1983). Psychotherapy for sexual deviation. *British Journal of Psychiatry, 143,* 242–247.

Davidmann, S. (2014). Imag(in)ing trans partnerships: Collaborative photography and intimacy. *Journal of Homosexuality, 61* (5), 636–653.

Davies, D., & Neal, C. (Eds.). (1996). *Pink therapy.* Maidenhead: The Open University Press.

Davis, N. Z. (1975). *Society and culture in early modern France: Eight essays.* Stanford, CA: Stanford University Press.

Davy, Z. (2008). Transsexual recognition: Embodiment bodily aesthetics and the medicolegal system. PhD thesis. Leeds: University of Leeds.

Davy, Z. (2010). Transsexual agents: Negotiating authenticity and embodiment in the UK's medicolegal system. In S. Hines & T. Sanger (Eds.), *Transgender identities: Towards an analysis of gender diversity* (pp. 106–126). Abingdon: Routledge.

Davy, Z. (2015). The DSM-5 and the politics of diagnosing transpeople. *Archives of Sexual Behavior, 44,* 1165–1176.

de Beauvoir, S. (1986 [1947]). *The ethics of ambiguity* [Trans B. Frechtman]. New York: Citadel Press.

de Beauvoir, S. (1997 [1949]). *The second sex* [Trans H. M. Parshley]. New York: Vintage.

de Cuypere, G. (1995). *Transseksualiteit: Psychiatrische aspecten in het kader van geslachtsaanpassende behandeling.* Proefschrift tot het verkrijgen van de graad van Doctor in de Biomedische Wetenschappen, Universiteit Gent.

de Cuypere, G., Van Hemelrijck, M., Michel, A., Carael, B., Heylens, G., Rubens, R., Hoebeke, P., & Monstrey, S. (2007). Prevalence and demography of transsexualism in Belgium. *European Psychiatry, 22,* 137–141.

Delcourt, M. (1961). Hermaphrodite: Myths and rites of the bisexual figure in classical antiquity [Trans J. Nicholson]. London: Studio Books.

De Roo, C., Tilleman, K., T'Sjoen, G., & De Sutter, P. (2016). Fertility options in transgender people. *International Review of Psychiatry, 28* (1), 112–119.

Derrida, J. (1998 [1967]). *Of grammatology* [Trans G. C. Spivak]. Baltimore, MA: Johns Hopkins University Press.

Diamond, M. (Ed.). (2011). Trans/love: Radical sex, love and relationships beyond the gender binary. San Francisco: Manic D Press.

Dickinson, T., Cook, M., Playle, J., & Hallett, C. (2012). 'Queer' treatments: Giving a voice to former patients who received treatments for their 'sexual deviations'. *Journal of Clinical Nursing, 21* (9–10), 1345–1354.

Doorduin, T., & Van Berlo, W. (2014). Trans people's experience of sexuality in the Netherlands: A pilot study. *Journal of Homosexuality, 61* (5), 654–672.

Dreger, A. D. (2008). The controversy surrounding the man who would be queen: A case history of the politics of science, identity, and sex in the internet age. *Archives of Sexual Behavior, 37* (3), 366–421.

Drescher, D. (2010). Queer diagnoses: Parallels and contrasts in the history of homosexuality, gender variance, and the diagnostic and statistical manual. *Archives of Sexual Behavior, 39* (2), 427–460.

du Plock, S. (2014 [1997]). Gay affirmative therapy: A critique and some reflections on the value of an existential-phenomenological theory of sexual identity. In M. Milton (Ed.), *Sexuality: Existential perspectives* (pp. 141–159). Ross-on-Wye: PCCS Books.

Easton, D., & Liszt, C. A. (1997). *The ethical slut*. San Francisco: Greenery Press.

Easton, D., & Hardy, J. W. (2001). *The new bottoming book*. San Francisco: Greenery Press.

Easton, D., & Hardy, J. W. (2002). *The new topping book*. San Francisco: Greenery Press.

Easton, D., & Hardy, J. W. (2005). *Radical ecstasy*. San Francisco: Greenery Press.

Ekins, R. (1997). *Male femaling*. London: Routledge.

Etherington, K. (2004). *Becoming a reflexive researcher*. London: Jessica Kingsley Publishers.

Ettner, R. (1999). *Gender loving care*. New York: Norton.

Ettner, R. (2007). Transsexual couples: A qualitative evaluation of atypical partner preferences. *International Journal of Transgenderism, 10* (2), 109–116.

Ettner, R., Monstrey, S., & Eyler, A. E. (Eds.). (2007). *Principles of transgender medicine and surgery*. New York: The Haworth Press.

Evans, J. L. (2011). *Genderqueer identity and self-perception*. (Dissertation) Alliant International University: San Francisco.

Farvid, P. (2015). Heterosexuality. In C. Richards & M. J. Barker (Eds.), *The Palgrave handbook of the psychology of sexuality and gender* (pp. 92–108). Basingstoke: Palgrave Macmillan.

Feinberg, L. (1993). *Stone butch blues*. New York: Firebrand Books.

Feinberg, L. (1996). *Transgender warriors*. Boston: Beacon Press.

Fenichel, O. (1930). The psychology of transvestitism. *International Journal of Psycho-Analysis, 11*, 211–227.

Finlay, L., & Gough, B. (2003). Reflexivity: A practical guide for researchers in health and social sciences. Oxford: Blackwell.

Firth, M. T. (2015). Childhood abuse, depressive vulnerability and gender dysphoria: Part 2. *Counselling and Psychotherapy Research, 15* (2), 98–108.

Fiske, S. T., & Taylor, S. E. (1991). *Social cognition* (2nd ed.). New York: McGraw-Hill Inc.

Forde, A. (2011). Evolutionary theory of mate selection and partners of trans people: A qualitative study using interpretative phenomenological analysis. *Qualitative Report, 16* (5), 1407–1434.

Foucault, M. (1991 [1977]). *Discipline and punish: The birth of the prison* (2nd ed.) [Trans A. Sheridan]. New York: Vintage Books.

Foucault, M. (1998 [1976]). *The history of sexuality, Vol. 1: The will to knowledge* [Trans R. Hurley]. London: Penguin Books Ltd.

Freegard, H. C. (2000). Living with a transvestite: A phenomenological study of wives and committed partners of transvestites. Doctoral thesis, Joondalup: Edith Cowan University.

Frith, H. (2000). Focusing on sex: Using focus groups in sex research. *Sexualities, 3* (3), 275–297.

Gadamer, H-G. (2004 [1960]). *Truth and method* (2nd ed.) [Trans J. Weinsheimer & D. G. Marshall]. New York: Crossroad.

Gagne, P., & Tewksbury, R. A. (2002). Introduction. In P. Gagne & R. A. Tewksbury (Eds.), *Gendered sexualities: Advances in gender research* (pp. 1–19). Boston, MA: JAI Press.

Garber, M. (1992). Vested interests: Cross-dressing and cultural anxiety. London: Penguin.

Garcia-Falgueras, A., & Swaab, D. (2008). A sex difference in the hypothalamic uncinate nucleus: Relationship to gender identity. *Brain, 131,* 3132–3146.

Gauntlett, D. (2007). *Creative explorations.* London: Routledge.

Gelder, M. G., & Marks, I. M. (1969). Aversion treatment in transvestism and transsexualism. In R. Green & J. Money (Eds.), *Transsexualism and sex reassignment* (pp. 383–413). Baltimore: The Johns Hopkins Press.

Giddens, A. (1984). *Social theory and modern sociology.* Cambridge: Polity Press.

Gijs, L., & Brewaeys, A. (2007). Surgical treatment of gender dysphoria in adults and adolescents: Recent developments, effectiveness, and challenges. *Annual Review of Sex Research, 18,* 178–224.

Gillespie, A., & Cornish, F. (2009). Intersubjectivity: Towards a dialogical analysis. *Journal for the Theory of Social Behaviour, 40* (1), 19–46.

Glaser, B. G., & Strauss, A. L. (1967). *The discovery of grounded theory: Strategies for qualitative research.* Chicago, IL: Aldine Publishing Co.

Gooren, L. J. G. (1984). Sexual dimorphism and transsexuality: Clinical observations. *Progress in Brain Research, 61,* 399–406.

Gooren, L. J. G. (1990). The endocrinology of transsexualism: A review and commentary. *Psychoneuroendocrinology, 15* (1), 3–14.

Green, J. (2004). *Becoming a visible man.* Nashville: Vanderbilt University Press.

Green, R. (2008). Lighten up, ladies. *Archives of Sexual Behavior, 37* (3), 451–452.

Green, R., & Money, J. (Eds.). (1969). *Transsexualism and sex reassignment.* Baltimore: The Johns Hopkins Press.

Habarta, N., Wang, G., Mulatu, M. S., & Larish, N. (2015). HIV testing by transgender status at Centers for Disease Control and Prevention – funded sites in the United States, Puerto Rico, and US Virgin Islands, 2009–2011. *American Journal of Public Health,* 105 (9):1917–1925.

Hagger-Johnson, G., Hegarty, P., Barker, M., & Richards, C. (2013). Public engagement, knowledge transfer, and impact validity. *Journal of Social Issues, 69* (4), 664–683.

Hall, K. (1995). Lip service on the fantasy lines. In K. Hall & M. Bucholtz (Eds.), *Gender articulated: Language and the socially constructed self* (pp. 183–216). New York: Routledge.

Haraldsen, I. R., & Dahl, A. A. (2000). Symptom profiles of gender dysphoric patients of transsexual type compared to patients with personality disorders and healthy adults. *Acta Psychiatrica Scandinavica, 102* (4), 276–281.

Harper, D. (2002). Talking about pictures: A case for photo elicitation. *Visual Studies, 17* (1), 13–26.

Harry Benjamin International Gender Dysphoria Association. (2001). *Standards of care* (6th ed.). Minneapolis, MN: World Professional Association for Transgender Health.

HCPC (Health and Care Professions Council). (2012). *Standards of proficiency: Practitioner psychologists*. London: Health Professions Council.

Heidegger, M. (2008 [1962]). *Being and time* (7th ed.) [Trans J. MacQuarrie & E. Robinson]. New York: Harper Collins.

Herbst, J. H., Jacobs, E. D., Finlayson, T. J., McKleroy, V. S., Neumann, M. S., & Crepaz, N. (2008). Estimating HIV prevalence and risk behaviors of transgender persons in the United States: A systematic review. *AIDS Behaviour, 12*, 1–17.

Herdt, G. (1996). *Third sex third gender*. New York: Zone books.

Hicks, C., & Milton, M. (2010). Sexual identities: Meanings for counselling psychology practice. In R. Woolfe., S. Strawbridge., B. Douglas., & W. Dryden (Eds.), *Handbook of counselling psychology* (pp. 257–275). London: Sage.

Hill, D. B., Rozanski, C., Carfagnini, J., & Willoughby, B. (2005). Gender identity disorders in childhood and adolescence: A critical inquiry. In D. Karasic & J. Drescher (Eds.), *Sexual and gender diagnoses of the diagnostic and statistical manual (DSM)* (pp. 7–34). New York: The Haworth Press.

Hines, S., & Sanger, T. (2010). Transgender identities: Towards a social analysis of gender diversity. New York: Routledge.

Hird, M. J. (2002a). Out/performing our selves: Invitation for dialogue. *Sexualities, 5* (3), 337–356.

Hird, M. J. (2002b). Welcoming dialogue: A further response to out/performing our selves. *Sexualities, 5* (3), 362–366.

Hirschfeld, M. (1938). *Sexual anomalies and perversions*. London: Encyclopaedic Press.

HMSO. (2004). Gender Recognition Act. London: HMSO.

HMSO. (2010). Single Equality Act. London: HMSO.

Hoekzema, E., Schagen, S. E. E., Kreukels, B. P. C., Veltman, D. J., Cohen-Kettenis, P. T., Delemarre-van de Waal, H., &, Bakker, J. (2015). Regional volumes and spatial volumetric distribution of gray matter in the gender dysphoric brain. *Psychoneuroendocrinology, 55*, 59–71.

Hofer, G. (1960). On the disguised person: A contribution to the phenomenology of transvestite behavior patterns. *Borderland of Psychiatry, 3*, 217–238.

Hoshiai, M., Matsumoto, Y., Sato, T., Ohnishi, M., Okabe, N., Kishimoto, Y., Terada, S., & Kuroda, S. (2010). Psychiatric comorbidity among patients with gender identity disorder. *Psychiatry and Clinical Neurosciences, 64*, 514–519.

Houghtaling, M. K. (2013). *Materiality, becoming and time: The existential phenomenology of sexuality*. Doctoral thesis, Queen's University, Kingston, Ontario, Canada.

Hoyer, N. (1933). Man into woman: An authentic record of a change of sex: The true story of the miraculous transformation of the Danish painter Einar Wegener-Andreas Sparre. London: Jarrolds.

Hunt, J. (2014). An initial study of transgender people's experiences of seeking and receiving counselling or psychotherapy in the UK. *Counselling and Psychotherapy research, 14* (4), 288–296.

Hunt, S., & Main, T. L. (1997). Sexual orientation confusion among spouses of transvestites and transsexuals following disclosure of spouse's gender dysphoria. *Journal of Psychology & Human Sexuality, 9* (2), 39–51.

Husserl, E. (1970 [1900]). *Logical investigations* [Trans J. N. Findlay]. New York: Humanities Press.

Husserl, E. (1973). On the phenomenology of intersubjectivity: Texts from the estate, Part 1: 1905–1920 (Zur Phänomenologie der intersubjektivität. Texte aus dem Nachlass. Erster Teil. 1905–1920). Edited by I. Kern. The Hague, the Netherlands: Martinus Nijhoff.

Iantaffi, A., & Bockting, W. O. (2011). Views from both sides of the bridge? Gender, sexual legitimacy and transgender people's experiences of relationships. *Culture, Health and Sexuality, 13* (3), 355–370.

Idso, E. L. (2009). A phenomenological exploration of transgender couples intimate relationships during transitioning: Implications for therapists. MSc Dissertation, Menomonie: University of Wisconsin-Stout.

Irigaray, L. (1985 [1977]). *This sex which is not one (Ce sexe qui n'en est pas un)* [Trans C. Porter & C. Burke]. New York: Cornell University Press.

Jorgensen, C. (1967). *A personal autobiography.* New York: Paul S Eriksson Inc.

Joseph, A. (2009). An inquiry into sexual difference in Ernesto Spinelli's psychology: An Irigarayan critique in response to Ernesto Spinelli's psychology. Saarbrüken: VDM Verlag.

Judd, D., & Milton, M. (2001). Psychotherapy with lesbian and gay clients: Existential-phenomenological contributions to training. *Lesbian and Gay Psychology Review, 2* (1), 16–23.

Junginger, J. (1997). Fetishism: Assessment and treatment. In D. R. Laws & W. O'Donohue (Eds.), *Sexual deviance: Theory assessment and treatment* (pp. 92–110). New York: Guildford Press.

Kahr, B. (1994). Sadomasochism and child sexual abuse – a response to Man Cheung Chung. *Journal of the Society for Existential Analysis, 5,* 121.

Kalraa, G., & Shahb, N. (2013). The cultural, psychiatric, and sexuality aspects of Hijras in India. *International Journal of Transgenderism, 14* (4), 171–181.

Karasic, D., & Drescher, J. (2005). Sexual and gender diagnoses of the diagnostic and statistical manual (DSM). New York: Haworth Press.

Kenagy, G. P., & Hsieh. C. M. (2005). The risk less known: Female-to-male transgender persons' vulnerability to HIV infection. *AIDS Care, 17* (2), 195–207.

Kersting, A., Reutemann, M., Gast, U., Ohrmann, P., Suslow, T., Michael, N., & Arolt, V. (2003). Dissociative disorders and traumatic childhood experiences in transsexuals. *Journal of Nervous and Mental Disease, 191* (3), 182–189.

Kidd, S. A., Veltman, A., Gately, C., Chan, K. J., & Cohen, J. N. (2011). Lesbian, gay, and transgender persons with severe mental illness: Negotiating wellness in the context of multiple sources of stigma. *American Journal of Psychiatric Rehabilitation, 14* (1), 13–39.

Kierkegaard, S. (1980 [1844]). *The concept of anxiety* [Trans R. Thomte & A. B. Anderson]. Princeton, NJ: Princeton University Press.

Kitzinger, J. (1994). The methodology of focus groups: The importance of interaction between research participants. *Sociology of Health and Illness, 16* (1), 103–121.

Kleinplatz, P. J., & Moser, C. (2005). Politics versus science: An addendum and response to Drs Spitzer and Fink. In D. Karasic & J. Drescher (Eds.), *Sexual and gender diagnoses of the diagnostic and statistical manual (DSM)* (pp. 91–109). New York: The Haworth Press.

Kosko, B. (1994). Fuzzy thinking: The new science of fuzzy logic. New York: Hyperion.

Krafft-Ebing, R. von. (1886). *Psychopathia sexualis: Eine klinisch-forensische studie* (Sexual psychopathy: A clinical-forensic study). Stuttgart: Ferdinand Enke.

Krafft-Ebing, R. von. (1906). *Psychopathia sexualis* (12th ed.). London: Rebman Ltd.

Krueger, R. B., & Kaplan, M. S. (2002). Behavioral and psychopharmacological treatment of the paraphilic and hypersexual disorders. *Journal of Psychiatric Practice, 8,* 21–32.

Kruijver, F. P. M. (2004). *Sex in the brain.* Amsterdam: Netherlands Institute of Brain Research.

Kruijver, F. P. M., Jiang-Ning, Z., Pool, C. W., Hofman, M. A., Gooren, L. J. G., & Swaab, D. F. (2000). Male-to-female transsexuals have female neuron numbers in a limbic nucleus. *The Journal of Clinical Endocrinology & Metabolism*, *85* (5), 2034–2041.

Langdridge, D. (2007). *Phenomenological psychology*. Harlow: Pearson.

Langdridge, D. (2013). *Existential counselling and psychotherapy*. London: Sage.

Langdridge, D. (2014). Gay affirmative therapy: Recognising the power of the social world. In M. Milton (Ed.), *Sexuality: Existential perspectives* (pp. 160–173). Monmouth: PCCS Books.

Langdridge, D., & Hagger-Johnson, G. (2009). *Introduction to research methods and data analysis in psychology* (2nd ed.). Harlow: Pearson Education.

Langer, S. J. (2011). Gender (dis)agreement: A dialogue on the clinical implications of gendered language. *Journal of Gay & Lesbian Mental Health*, *15* (3), 300–307.

Lawrence, A. A. (2005). Sexuality after male-to-female sex reassignment surgery. *Archives of Sexual Behaviour*, *34* (2), 147–166.

Lawrence, A. A. (2013). *Men trapped in men's bodies: Narratives of autogynephilic transsexualism*. New York, NY: Springer.

Laws, D. R. (2001). Olfactory aversion: Notes on procedure, with speculations on its mechanism of effect. *Sex Abuse*, *13* (4), 275–287.

Leighton, T. (1999). Existential freedom and political change. In J. S. Murphy (Ed.), *Feminist interpretations of Jean-Paul Sartre* (pp. 149–173). University Park: Pennsylvania State University Press.

Lenihan, P., Kainth, T., & Dundas, R. (2015). Trans sexualities. In C. Richards & M. J. Barker (Eds.), *The Palgrave handbook of the psychology of sexuality and gender* (pp. 129–146). Basingstoke: Palgrave.

Lev, A. I. (2006). Disordering Gender Identity Disorder in the DSM-IV-TR. *Journal of Psychology & Human Sexuality*, *17* (3–4), 35–69.

Lev, A. I. (forthcoming, 2017). *Transgender emergence* (2nd ed.). London: Haworth Clinical Practice Press.

Levine, S. B. (2014). What is more bizarre: The transsexual or transsexual politics? *Sex Roles*, *70* (3–4), 158–160.

Levitt, H. M., & Ippolito, M. R. (2014). Being transgender navigating minority stressors and developing authentic self-presentation. *Psychology of Women Quarterly*, *38* (1), 46–64.

Lombardi, E. (2001). Enhancing transgender health care. *American Journal of Public Health*, *91* (6), 869–872.

Lombardi, E. L., Wilchins, R. A., Priesing, D., & Malouf, D. (2001). Gender violence: Transgender experiences with violence and discrimination. *Journal of Homosexuality*, *42* (1), 89–101.

Luft, J., & Ingham, H. (1955). The johari window: A graphic model of interpersonal awareness. In J. Luft (Ed.) (1969), *Of human interaction* (p. 177). Paolo Alto, CA. National Press.

Lyotard, J-F. (1984). *The postmodern condition: A report on knowledge* [Trans G. Bennington & B. Massumi]. Manchester: Manchester University Press.

Maher, A. L. (2011). The use of art and interview to explore the transgender person's experience of gender transition: A phenomenological study. Master's dissertation, Drexel University, Philadelphia.

Manafi, E. (2014). Foreword. In M. Milton (Ed.), *Sexuality: Existential perspectives* (pp. ix–xii–75). Monmouth: PCCS Books.

Marks, I. M., & Gelder, M. G. (1967). Transvestism and fetishism: Clinical and psychological changes during faradic aversion. *British Journal of Psychiatry*, *113*, 711–729.

Marks, I. M., Rachman, S., & Gelder, M. G. (1965). Methods for assessment of aversion treatment in fetishism with masochism. *Behaviour Research and Therapy, 3*, 253–258.

Martino, M., & Harriett. (1977). *Emergence: A transsexual autobiography.* New York: Crown Publishers Inc.

Mc Geeney, E., & Harvey, L. (2015). Cisgender. In C. Richards & M. J. Barker (Eds.), *The Palgrave handbook of the psychology of sexuality and gender* (pp. 149–165). Basingstoke: Palgrave Macmillan.

McNeil, J., Bailey, L., Ellis, S., Morton, J., & Regan, M. (2012). *Trans mental health survey 2012.* Edinburgh: Scottish Transgender Alliance.

McParland, J. L., & Flowers, P. (2012). Nine lessons and recommendations from the conduct of focus group research in chronic pain samples. *British Journal of Health Psychology, 17,* 492–504.

Medina, M. (2008). Can I be a homosexual please? A critique of sexual deliberations on the issue of homosexuality and their significance for the practice of existential psychotherapy. *Existential Analysis, 19* (1), 129–142.

Merleau-Ponty, M. (1996 [1945]). *Phenomenology of perception* [Trans C. Smith]. London: Routledge.

Merleau-Ponty, M. (2002 [1945]). *Phenomenology of perception* [Trans C. Smith]. London: Routledge.

Merton, R. K., Fiske, M., & Kendall, P. L. (1990). *The focused interview: A manual of problems and procedures* (2nd ed.). New York: Free Press.

Meyer, I. H. (1995). Minority stress and mental health in gay men. *Journal of Health and Social Behavior, 36,* 38–56.

Meyer-Bahlburg, H. F. (2010). From mental disorder to iatrogenic hypogonadism: Dilemmas in conceptualizing gender identity variants as psychiatric conditions. *Archives of Sexual Behavior, 39* (2), 461–476.

Meyerowitz, J. (2002). How sex changed: A history of transsexuality in the United States. London: Harvard University Press.

Milton, M. (1997). Is existential psychotherapy a lesbian and gay affirmative psychotherapy? *Journal of the Society for Existential Analysis, 11* (1), 86–102.

Milton, M. (2005). Political and ideological issues. In E. van Deurzen & C. Penhallow (Eds.), *Existential perspectives on human issues: A handbook for therapeutic practice.* (pp. 245–252) Basingstoke: Palgrave Macmillan.

Milton, M. (2007). Being sexual: Existential contributions to psychotherapy with gay male clients. In E. Peel., V. Clarke., & J. Drescher (Eds.), *British lesbian, gay and bisexual psychologies: Theory, research and practice.* (pp. 183–198) Binghampton, NY: The Haworth Medical Press.

Milton, M. (2014a). Sexuality: Where existential thought and counselling psychology practice come together. *Counselling Psychology Review, 29* (2), 15–24.

Milton, M. (Ed.). (2014b). *Sexuality: Existential perspectives.* Ross-on-Wye: PCCS Books.

Milton, M. (2014c). Sexuality: Debates and controversies. In M. Milton (Ed.), *Sexuality: Existential perspectives* (pp. 1–18). Monmouth: PCCS Books.

Milton, M., & Coyle, A. (2003). Sexual identity: Affirmative practice with lesbian and gay clients. In R. Woolfe., S. Strawbridge., & W. Dryden (Eds.), *Handbook of counselling psychology* (2nd ed.) (pp. 481–499). London: Sage.

Minton, H. L. (2002). Departing from deviance: A history of homosexual rights and emancipatory science in America. Chicago, IL: University of Chicago Press.

Moon. L. (Ed.). (2008). *Feeling queer or queer feelings?: Radical approaches to counselling sex, sexualities and genders.* Hove: Routledge.

Money, J., Hampson, J. G., & Hampson, J. L. (1957). Imprinting and the establishment of gender role. *Archives of Neurology and Psychiatry, 77*, 333–336.

Morgan, D. L. (1997). *Focus groups as qualitative research* (2nd ed.). Thousand Oaks: Sage Publications.

Morgan, D. L., & Ruszczynski, S. (Eds.). (2006). *Lectures on violence perversion and delinquency.* London: Karnac.

Morris, J. (1974). *Conundrum: From James to Jan: An extraordinary personal narrative of transsexualism.* New York: Harcourt Brace Jovanovich.

Moser, C. (2009). Autogynephilia in women. *Journal of Homosexuality, 56* (5), 539–547.

Moustakas, C. (1994). *Phenomenological research methods.* London: Sage.

Mukaddes, N. M. (2002). Gender identity problems in autistic children. *Child: Care, Health and Development, 28*, 529–532.

Murjan, S., & Bouman, W. P. (2015). Trans gender. In C. Richards & M. Barker (Eds.), *The Palgrave handbook of the psychology of sexuality and gender.* (pp.198–215). Basingstoke: Palgrave Macmillan.

Myers, G. (1998). Displaying opinions: Topics and disagreement in focus groups. *Language in Society, 27*, 85–111.

Naylor, G. [Writer]., & May, J., Grant, R., & Naylor, D. [Directors]. (1992). *The inquisitor* [Television series episode]. In Grant, R., & Naylor, D. [Producers], Red Dwarf. London: British Broadcasting Corporation.

Neal, C., & Davies, D. (Eds.). (2000). *Issues in therapy with lesbian, gay, bisexual and transgender clients.* Maidenhead: Open University Press.

Nemoto, T., Operario, D., Keatley, J., & Villegas, D. (2004). Social context of HIV risk behaviours among male-to-female transgenders of colour. *AIDS Care, 16* (6), 724–735.

NHS Calderdale. (2009). *Survey of the trans population in Calderdale.* Retrieved 7 June 2013 from: www.calderdale.nhs.uk/fileadmin/files/Public_Information/Publications/Microsoft_ Word_-_Calderdale_Trans_Report_-_March__09.pdf

NHS Citizen. (2015). *NHS citizen assembly stocktake (March 2015): Gender identity services.* Retrieved 9 June from: www.nhscitizen.org.uk/wp-content/uploads/2015/03/Gender-ID.pdf

NHS England. (2013). Interim gender dysphoria protocol and service guideline 2013/14. London: NHS England.

Nietzsche, F. (1882). *Die fröhliche wissenschaft (The gay science).* Leipzig: Verlag von E. W. Fritzsch.

Nietzsche, F. (1968 [1895]). *The will to power (der wille zur macht)* [Trans W. Kaufmann & R. J. Hollingdale]. New York: Vintage Books.

Orlans, V., & Van Scoyoc, S. (2009). *A short introduction to counselling psychology.* London: Sage.

Owen, I. R. (2012). The phenomenological psychology of gender: How trans-sexuality and intersexuality express the general case of self as a cultural object. *Phaenomenologica, 199*, 199–212.

Oxford Dictionaries. (2015a). *Sexuality.* Retrieved 8 June 2015 from: www.oxforddictionaries. com/definition/english/sexuality

Oxford Dictionaries. (2015b). *Sexual.* Retrieved 8 June 2015 from: www.oxforddictionaries. com/definition/english/sexuality

Parsons, M., & Greenwood, J. (2000). A guide to the use of focus groups in healthcare research: Part 1. *Contemporary Nursing, 9* (2), 169–180.

Pearce, R. (2011). Escaping into the other: An existential view of sex and sexuality. *Existential Analysis, 22* (2), 229–243.

Pearce, R. (2014). Sexual expression: Authenticity and bad faith. In M. Milton (Ed.), *Sexuality: Existential perspectives* (pp. 92–115). Monmouth: PCCS Books Ltd.

Person, E., & Ovesey, L. (1974). The transsexual syndrome in males: I. Primary transsexualism. *American Journal of Psychotherapy, 28*, 4–29.

Plummer, K. (1995). *Telling sexual stories: Power, change and social worlds*. New York: Routledge.

Pratchett, T. (1998). *Carpe jugulum*. London: Doubleday.

Prince, V. (1971). *How to be a woman though male*. Los Angeles, CA: Chevalier Publications.

Queen, C., & Schimel, L. (Eds.). (1997). *PoMoSexuals*. San Francisco: Cleis Press Inc.

Raymond, J. G. (1979). *The transsexual empire: The making of the she-male*. Boston: Beacon Press.

Raymond, M. J. (1956). Case of fetishism treated by aversion therapy. *British Medical Journal, 2*, 854–857.

Raymond, M. J. (1969). Aversion therapy for sexual perversions. *British Journal of Psychiatry, 115*, 979–980.

RCP (Royal College of Psychiatrists). (2013). *CR181 good practice guidelines for the assessment and treatment of gender dysphoria*. London: Royal College of Psychiatrists.

Reavey, P. (Ed.). (2011). *Visual psychologies: Using and interpreting images in qualitative research*. London: Routledge.

Reavey, P., & Johnson, K. (2008). Visual approaches: Using and interpreting images in qualitative research. In C. Willig & W. Stainton Rogers (Eds.), *The Sage handbook of qualitative research methods* (pp. 296–315). London: Sage.

Reed, B., Rhodes, S., Schofield, P., & Wylie, K. (2011). *Gender variance in the UK: Prevalence, incidence, growth and geographic distribution*. London: GIRES.

Rees, M. (1996). *Dear sir or madam: The autobiography of a female-to-male transsexual*. London: Cassell.

Rich, A. (1980). Compulsory heterosexuality and lesbian existence. *Signs, 5* (4), 631–660.

Richards, C. (2007). [Letter to the editor] Diagnosis under fire. *The Psychologist, 20* (7), 413.

Richards, C. (2010). Trans and non-monogamies. In D. Langdridge and M. Barker (Eds.), *Understanding non-monogamies* (pp. 121–133). London: Routledge.

Richards, C. (2011a). Are you sitting comfortably? Reader Injunctions: An addition to the methodologies of the human and natural sciences. *The Psychologist, 24* (12), 904–906.

Richards, C. (2011b). Transsexualism and existentialism. *Existential Analysis, 22* (2), 272–279.

Richards, C. (2014a). Trans and existentialism. In M. Milton (Ed.), *Existential perspectives* (pp. 217–230). Ross-on-Wye: PCCS Books.

Richards, C. (2014b). Group therapy and sexuality. In M. Milton (Ed.), *Sexuality: Existential perspectives* (pp. 265–284). Ross-on-Wye: PCCS Books.

Richards, C. (2015). Further sexualities. In C. Richards, & M. J. Barker (Eds.), *The Palgrave handbook of the psychology of sexuality and gender* (pp. 60–76). London: Palgrave-Macmillan.

Richards, C. (2016). Third genders: The Wiley-Blackwell encyclopedia of gender and sexuality studies. Hoboken, NJ: Wiley-Blackwell.

Richards, C. (2017a). *Publications*. Retrieved 27 January 2017 from: http://christinarichardspsychologist.wordpress.com/publications/

Richards, C. (2017b). Researching trans people: Ethics through method. In A. Porrovecchio, T. Claes, & P. Reynolds (Eds.), *Methodological and ethical issues in sex and sexuality research: Contemporary essays*. Leverkusen: Budrich Academic.

Richards, C. (2017c). Starshine on the critical edge: Philosophy and psychotherapy in fantasy and sci-fi. *Journal of Psychotherapy and Counselling Psychology Reflections, 2* (1), 17–24.

Richards, C., & Barker, M. J. (2013). Sexuality and gender for mental health professionals: A practical guide. London: Sage.

Richards, C., & Barker, M. J. (2015). *The Palgrave handbook of the psychology of sexuality and gender*. Basingstoke: Palgrave Macmillan.

Richards, C., Barker, M., Lenihan, P., & Iantaffi, A. (2014). Who watches the watchmen?: A critique on the theorization of trans people and clinicians. *Feminism and Psychology, 24* (2), 248–258.

Richards, C., Bouman, W. P., & Barker, M. (Eds.). (2017). *Genderqueer and non-binary genders.* London: Palgrave-Macmillan.

Richards, C., Bouman, W. P., Seal, L., Barker, M. J., Nieder, T., & T'Sjoen, G. (2016). Non-binary or genderqueer genders. *International Review of Psychiatry, 28* (1), 95–102.

Richards, C., & Lenihan, P. (2012). A critique of trans people's partnerships: Towards an ethics of intimacy by Tam Sanger. *Sexual and Relationship Therapy, 27* (1), 63–68.

Richards, C., & Seal, L. (2014). Reproductive issues for trans people. *BMJ, Journal of Family Planning and Reproductive Health Care, 40* (4), 245–247. doi:10.1136/jfprhc-2013-100669

Ricoeur, P. (1970). *Freud and philosophy: An essay on interpretation* [Trans D. Savage]. New Haven, CT: Yale University Press.

Ricoeur, P. (1984). *Time and narrative* (Vol. 1) [Trans K. McLaughlin & D. Pellauer]. Chicago, IL: New Haven Press: University of Chicago Press.

Ricoeur, P. (1985). *Time and narrative* (Vol. 2) [Trans K. McLaughlin & D. Pellauer]. Chicago, IL: New Haven Press: University of Chicago Press.

Ricoeur, P. (1988). *Time and narrative* (Vol. 3) [Trans K. McLaughlin & D. Pellauer]. Chicago, IL: New Haven Press: University of Chicago Press.

Robles, R., Fresán, A., Vega-Ramírez, H., Cruz-Islas, J., Rodríguez-Pérez, V., Domínguez-Martínez, T., & Reed, G. M. (2016). Removing transgender identity from the classification of mental disorders: A Mexican field study for ICD-11. *The Lancet Psychiatry, 3* (9), 850–859.

Rodrigues, V. A. (2014). Are sexual preferences existential choices? *Existential Analysis, 25,* (1), 43–52.

Rowniak, S., & Chesla, C. (2013). Coming out for a third time: Transmen, sexual orientation, and identity. *Archives of Sexual Behavior, 42* (3), 449–461.

Royal College of Psychiatrists (RCP). (2013). *CR181 good practice guidelines for the assessment and treatment of gender dysphoria*. London: Royal College of Psychiatrists.

Rubin, H. S. (1998). Phenomenology as method in trans studies. *Gay and Lesbian Quarterly, 4* (2), 263–281.

Rubin, H. S. (2003). *Self-made men: Identity and embodiment among transsexual men*. Nashville: Vanderbilt University Press.

Ruppin, U., & Pfafflin, F. (2015). Long-term follow-up of adults with Gender Identity Disorder. *Archives of Sexual Behavior, 44* (5), 1321–1329. doi: 10.1007/s10508-014-0453-5

Rutherford, K., McIntyre, J., Daley, A., & Ross, L. E. (2012). Development of expertise in mental health service provision for lesbian, gay, bisexual and transgender communities. *Medical Education, 46* (9), 903–913.

Salamon, G. (2010). *Assuming a body: Transgender and rhetorics of materiality*. New York: Columbia University Press.

Sanger, T. (2010). *Trans people's partnerships: Towards an ethics of intimacy*. Basingstoke: Palgrave.

Saraswat, A., Weinand, J. D., & Safer, J. D. (2015). Evidence supporting the biologic nature of gender identity. *Endocrine Practice, 21* (2), 199–204.

Sartre, J-P. (1996 [1943]). *Being and nothingness* [Trans H. E. Burns]. London: Routledge.

Sartre, J-P. (2003 [1943]). *Being and nothingness* [Trans H. E. Burns]. London: Routledge.

Saussure, F. de. (1916). *Cours de linguistique générale*. Edited by C. Bally & A. Sechehaye with the collaboration of A. Riedlinger. Paris: Payot.

Scarpella, K. M. (2011). Male-to-female transsexual individuals' experience of clinical relationships: A phenomenological study. Thesis, Ann Arbour, University of Michigan.

Schilt, K. (2010). *Just one of the guys? Transgender men and the persistence of gender inequality.* Chicago, IL: University of Chicago Press.

Schilt, K., & Windsor, E. (2014). The sexual habitus of transgender men: Negotiating sexuality through gender. *Journal of Homosexuality, 61* (5), 732–748.

Schlonski, D., & Adams, J. M. (1997). *The last time I wore a dress.* New York: Riverhead Books.

Schmich, M. (1997 June 1). *Advice, like youth, probably just wasted on the young.* Chicago, IL. Chicago Tribune. Retrieved 26 March 2014 from: www.chicagotribune.com/news/columnists/chi-schmich-sunscreencolumn,0,4054576.column?page=1

Segal, M. M. (1965). Transvestism as an impulse and as a defence. *International Journal of Psychoanalysis, 46,* 209–217.

Self, W., & Gamble, D. (2000). *Perfidious man.* London: Viking.

Serano, J. M. (2007). *Whipping girl.* Emeryville: Seal Press.

Serano, J. M. (2008). A matter of perspective: A transsexual woman-centric critique of Dreger's 'Scholarly History' of the Bailey controversy. *Archives of Sexual Behaviour, 37,* 491–494.

Serano, J. M. (2010). The case against autogynephilia. *International Journal of Transgenderism, 12* (3), 176–187.

Serning, N. (2012). Towards the cybernetic mind. *Existential Analysis, 23* (1), 7–14.

Shepherd, L. J., & Sjoberg, L. (2012). Trans-bodies in/of war(s): Cisprivilege and contemporary security strategy. *Feminist Review, 101,* 5–23.

Sherif, M. (1956). Experiments in group conflict. *Scientific American, 195,* 54–58.

Silverman, H. J. (1984). Phenomenology: From hermeneutics to deconstruction. *Research in Phenomenology, 14* (1), 19–34.

Simon, L., Zsolt, U., Fogd, D., & Czobor, P. (2011). Dysfunctional core beliefs, perceived parenting behavior and psychopathology in gender identity disorder: A comparison of male-to-female, female-to-male transsexual and nontranssexual control subjects. *Journal of Behavior Therapy and Experimental Psychiatry, 42* (1), 38–45.

Singer, B. (2013). The human simulation lab-dissecting sex in the simulator lab: The clinical lacuna of transsexed embodiment. *Journal of Medical Humanities, 34* (2), 249–254.

Smith, J. A. (2008). *Qualitative psychology.* London: Sage.

Smith, J. A. (2013). Unsettling the privilege of self reflexivity. In F. W. Twine & B. Gardener (Eds.), *Geographies of privilege* (pp. 263–280). New York: Routledge.

Smith Pickard, P. (2014) Merleau-Ponty and Existential Sexuality. In M. Milton (Ed.). *Sexuality Existential Perspectives.* (pp. 79–91) Ross-on-Wye: PCCS Books.

Spinelli, E. (1996). Some hurried notes expressing outline ideas that someone might someday utilise as signposts towards a sketch of an existential-phenomenological theory of sexuality. *Existential Analysis, 8* (1), 2–20.

Spinelli, E. (2007). Practicing existential psychotherapy: The relational world. London: Sage.

Spinelli, E. (2013). Being sexual: Human sexuality revisited: Part 1. *Existential Analysis, 24* (2), 297–317.

Spinelli, E. (2014). Being sexual: Human sexuality revisited: Part 2. *Existential Analysis, 25* (1), 17–42.

Stewart, D. W., & Shamdasani, P. M. (1990). *Focus groups: Theory and practice.* Newbury Park, CA: Sage.

Stryker, S. (2008). Dungeon intimacies: The poetics of transsexual sadomasochism. *Parallax, 14* (1), 36–47.

Stoller, R. J. (1964). A contribution to the study of gender identity. *International Journal of Psychoanalysis, 45*, 220–226.

Stryker, S., & Whittle, S. (Eds.). (2006). *The transgender studies reader.* London: Routledge.

Sue, D. W. (2010). *Microaggressions in everyday life: Race, gender and sexual orientation.* Hoboken: Wiley.

Suzuki, S. (2011 [1970]). *Zen mind, beginner's mind.* Boston, MA: Shambhala Publications Inc.

Swaab, D. F., & Garcia-Falgueras, A. (2008). Sexual differentiation of the human brain in relation to gender identity and sexual orientation. *Functional Neurology, 24*, 17–28.

Taormino, T. (2012). *Ultimate guide to kink.* San Francisco: Cleis Press Inc.

Tompkins, A. B. (2014). 'There's no chasing involved': Cis/trans relationships, 'tranny chasers,' and the future of a sex-positive trans politics. *Journal of Homosexuality, 61* (5), 766–780.

Tosh, J. (2011). Challenging queerphobic practice: Protesting professor Ken Zucker's 'prevention' of gender diversity. *Psychology of Sexualities Review, 2* (1), 54–61.

Towle, E. B., & Morgan, L. M. (2006). Romancing the transgender native: Rethinking the use of the 'third gender' concept. In S. Stryker & S. Whittle (Eds.), *The transgender studies reader* (pp. 666–684). London: Routledge.

T'Sjoen, G., Van Caenegem, E., & Wierckx, K. (2013). Transgenderism and reproduction. *Current Opinion in Endocrinology, Diabetes and Obesity, 20* (6), 575–579.

Tsoi, W. F. (1988). The prevalence of transsexualism in Singapore. *Acta Psychiatrica Scandinavica, 78*, 501–504.

Vance Jr, S. R., Cohen-Kettenis, P. T., Drescher, J., Meyer-Bahlburg, H. F., Pfäfflin, F., & Zucker, K. J. (2010). Opinions about the DSM Gender Identity Disorder diagnosis: Results from an international survey administered to organizations concerned with the welfare of transgender people. *International Journal of Transgenderism, 12* (1), 1–14.

van Deurzen, E., & Adams, M. (2011). *Skills in existential counselling and psychotherapy.* London: Sage.

van Deurzen-Smith, E. (1997). *Everyday mysteries: Existential dimensions of psychotherapy.* London: Routledge.

van Manen, M. (1997). *Researching lived experience: Human science for an action sensitive pedagogy* (2nd ed.). London, Western Ontario: The Althouse Press.

van Manen, M. (2014). *Phenomenology of practice: Meaning giving methods in phenomenological research and writing.* Walnut Creek, CA: Left Coast Press Inc.

Veale, J. F. (2008). The prevalence of transsexualism among New Zealand passport holders. *Australian and New Zealand Journal of Psychiatry, 42* (10), 887–889.

Veale, J. F., Clarke, D. E., & Lomax, T. C. (2008). Sexuality of male-to-female transsexuals. *Archives of Sexual Behavior, 37* (4), 586–597.

Von Mahlsdorf, C. (1995 [1992]). *I am my own woman: The outlaw life of Charlotte Von Mahlsdorf, Berlin's most distinguished transvestite* (Ich bin meine eigene frau) [Trans J. Hollander]. San Francisco: Cleis Press.

Wallien, M. S., Zucker, K. J., Steensma, T. D., & Cohen-Kettenis, P. T. (2008). 2D:4D finger-length ratios in children and adults with gender identity disorder. *Hormones and Behavior, 54* (3), 450–454.

Warner, M. (2000). *The trouble with normal: Sex, politics, and the ethics of queer life.* Cambridge, MA: Harvard University Press.

Weeks, J. (1999). *Making sexual history.* Cambridge: Polity Press.

Weeks, J. (2007). *The world we have won: The remaking of erotic and intimate life* (New ed.). London: Routledge.

Weinberg, M. S., & Williams, C. J. (2010). Men sexually interested in transwomen (MSTW): Gendered embodiment and the construction of sexual desire. *Journal of Sex Research, 47* (4), 374–383.

Weyers, S., Elaut, E., De Suter, P., Gerris, J., T'Sjoen, G., Heylens, G., De Cuypere, G., & Verstraelen, H. (2009). Long term assessment of the physical, mental and sexual health among transsexual women. *Journal of Sexual Medicine, 6* (3), 752–760.

Widdowson, M. (2012). Perceptions of psychotherapy trainees of psychotherapy research. *Counselling and Psychotherapy Research, 13,* 176–186.

Wilchins, R. A. (1997). *Read my lips: Sexual subversion and the end of gender.* Ann Arbor: Firebrand Books.

Wilkinson, S. (2008). Focus groups. In J. A. Smith (Ed.), *Qualitative psychology: A practical guide to research methods* (2nd ed.) (pp. 186–206). London: Sage.

Wilson, C. K., West, L., Stepleman, L., Villarosa, M., Ange, B., Decker, M., & Waller, J. L. (2014). Attitudes toward LGBT patients among students in the health professions: Influence of demographics and discipline. *LGBT Health, 1* (3), 204–211.

Wilson, P., Sharp, C., & Carr, S. (1999). The prevalence of gender dysphoria in Scotland: A primary care study. *British Journal of General Practice, 49* (449), 991–992.

Wilton, T. (2002). 'You think this song is about you': Reply to Hird. *Sexualities, 5* (3), 357–361.

Windsor, E. J. (2006). *Getting by gatekeepers: Transmen's dialectical negotiations within psychomedical institutions.* Unpublished thesis, Atlanta, Georgia State University, Department of Sociology.

Winters, K., & Ehrbar, R. D. (2010). Beyond conundrum: Strategies for diagnostic harm reduction. *Journal of Gay & Lesbian Mental Health, 14* (2), 130–138.

Woolfe, R., Dryden, W., & Strawbridge, S. (Eds.). (2003). *Handbook of counselling psychology* (2nd ed.). London: Sage.

World Health Organization. (1965). *International Classification of Diseases 8.* Geneva: WHO.

World Health Organization. (1992). *International Classification of Diseases 10* (2nd ed.). Geneva: WHO.

World Professional Association for Transgender Health (WPATH). (2011). *Standards of care for the heath of transsexual, transgender and gender nonconforming people* (7th ed.). Minneapolis, MN: WPATH.

Zhou, J. N., Hofman, M. A., Gooren, L. J., & Swaab, D. F. (1995). A sex difference in the human brain and its relation to transsexuality. *Nature, 378,* 68–70.

Zucker, K. J., Bradley, S. J., Owen-Anderson, A., Kibblewhite, S. J., Wood, H., Singh, D., & Choi, K. (2012). Demographics, behavior problems, and psychosexual characteristics of adolescents with gender identity disorder or transvestic fetishism. *Journal of Sex & Marital Therapy, 38* (2), 151–189.

The doctoral thesis upon which this monograph was based was undertaken at the New School of Counselling and Psychotherapy Ltd and accredited by Middlesex University.

Index

International Classification of Diseases (ICD)
    1, 2, 5n4, 12, 13, 34
internet 15, 20, 25, 44, 71, 72, 89, 96, 128
intersection 3, 40, 66
intersex 20, 30

kink 31, 57, 73, 74, 76, 83, 91, 129, 131, 133,
    135, 137; see also BDSM

label 19, 28, 29, 40, 46, 53, 54, 59, 61, 69, 79,
    83, 90, 91, 95, 101, 102, 106, 107, 108
language 4, 16, 39, 45, 61, 62, 90, 91, 94, 95,
    101, 103, 130, 134
leather 31, 58, 59, 63, 64, 83, 90, 91
legal 24, 42, 43, 56, 95
LEGO 34, 36, 45, 58, 63, 74, 89, 91, 95, 101,
    103, 108n1
lesbian 18, 26, 30n17, 95, 130, 131, 133, 135
LGBT – Lesbian Gay Bisexual Transgender
    Queer (LGBTQ)/LG/LGB/LGBT etc. 28
loss 43, 80
lower surgery 81, 83, 84, 85

mainstream 36, 38, 129, 134, 135, 136
male ii, 1, 5n3, 8, 9, 10, 11, 13, 14, 19, 24, 25,
    28, 29, 30n6, 46, 47, 53, 54, 60, 61, 62, 66,
    68, 74, 75, 76, 78, 81, 82, 83, 85, 87, 90, 91,
    92, 95, 107, 126, 127, 128, 130, 135, 136
male to female (MtF) 74, 75, 76, 82, 91, 128;
    see also trans woman
man 5n3, 15, 16, 24, 25, 26, 30n9, 46, 47,
    53, 54, 58, 62, 64, 65, 74, 81, 83, 87, 89,
    91, 101, 102, 107, 136, 142n1
masculine 57, 58, 59, 74, 76, 78, 81, 82, 102,
    127, 136
masculinity 8, 25, 58, 59, 60, 62, 73, 74, 75,
    76, 78, 81, 82, 90, 134, 136
masturbation 12, 69
media 34, 54, 71, 95, 126, 129, 135
medical i, 11, 12, 15, 18, 24, 80, 81, 87, 89,
    125, 126, 130
medicine 3, 8, 11, 12, 24
mental health ii, iv, 4, 5, 15, 21, 46
man who has sex with men (MSM) 102
metoidioplasty 84, 88, 90
minority ii, 12, 41, 62, 93, 128
minority/marginalisation stress 12, 105
moral 12, 42
multidisciplinary ii

name 8, 18, 59, 61, 69, 71, 72, 91, 135
natural 12, 29
negotiate 22, 76
neutrois 2, 47n5

normal 13, 73, 122
nymphomania 12

one, the 13, 50, 74, 75, 85
online 71, 72, 96, 98, 104, 128, 134
orgasm 20
orientation 3, 22, 28, 35, 53, 59, 83
other ii, vi, 1, 3, 5n9, 6, 8, 9, 11, 17, 19, 20, 21,
    24, 27, 28, 29, 30n6, 37, 38, 41, 44, 46, 51,
    53, 56, 57, 59, 61, 64, 66, 68, 71, 72, 74, 78,
    82, 85, 87, 90, 91, 93, 95, 96, 100, 101, 102,
    104
out 4, 6, 8, 12, 21, 25, 28, 31, 36, 42, 44, 45,
    53, 61, 62, 71, 72, 81, 96, 97, 100, 102, 103,
    104, 106, 107, 138

pain 39
pansexual 57, 82
paraphilia 12
parents 14
parties 18, 21
partner 22, 25, 28, 65, 76, 83, 85, 137
partnered sex 28
passive 4, 103
pass/passing 38, 39, 45, 74, 95, 127
penis 78, 83, 84, 92n10, 103, 107, 136
phenomenology 3, 4, 6, 7, 21, 27, 32, 33, 34,
    35, 38, 39, 106
physiology 30n10
play 21, 56, 68, 83, 86
polyamory/poly 18, 46, 47n8, 83, 129
postmodern 17, 25, 26, 53, 58, 59, 64, 75, 107,
    108
power 8, 53, 59, 64, 74, 75, 76, 86, 91n4, 95,
    97, 106, 108
prejudice 105
primary care 11, 43
privilege 74, 75, 76, 89, 103
psychiatric i, 1, 10, 12, 13, 81, 89
psychiatrist 88, 89
psychoanalysis 42, 106
psychologist ii, x, 3, 4, 8, 11, 15, 16, 17, 18, 21,
    23, 41, 51, 53, 56, 87, 100, 101, 102, 105,
    106, 107, 108
psychology i, ii, iv, v, 3, 6, 11, 16, 17, 24, 38,
    40, 54, 61, 66
psychopathology 11, 12, 13
psychotherapist i, ii, 16, 26, 93
psychotherapy i, ii
puberty 68, 82

qualitative i, 20, 31, 32, 41, 69, 96
quantitative ix, 20, 31, 32, 69, 125
queen 138